Radiographic Imaging & Exposure

Radiographic
&Imaging
Exposure

Terri L. Fauber, Ed.D., R.T. (R)(M)

Chair and Assistant Professor
Department of Radiation Sciences
Virginia Commonwealth University/
Medical College of Virginia Campus
Richmond, Virginia

with 265 illustrations

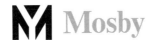 Mosby

A Harcourt Health Sciences Company

St. Louis   Philadelphia   London   Sydney   Toronto

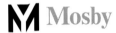

A Harcourt Health Sciences Company

Executive Editor: Jeanne Wilke
Associate Developmental Editor: Jennifer Genett
Developmental Editor: Carole Glauser
Project Manager: Carol Sullivan Weis
Project Specialist: Pat Joiner
Book Design Manager: Judi Lang
Cover Designer: Kathi Gosche
Interior Designer: Brian Salisbury

Mosby, Inc.
A Harcourt Health Sciences Company
11830 Westline Industrial Drive
St. Louis, Missouri 63146

Printed in the United States of America

Library of Congress Cataloging in Publication Data

Fauber, Terri L.
    Radiographic imaging and exposure / Terri L. Fauber.
       p. cm
    Includes index.
    ISBN 0-323-00405-9
    1. Radiography, Medical—Exposure. 2. Radiography, Medical—Image quality. I. Title.
    RC78 .F33 2000
    616.07´572—dc21
                                                                                            99-089531

00 01 02 03 04 GW/FF 9 8 7 6 5 4 3 2 1

Eugene D. Frank, M.A., R.T.(R) FASRT
Director, Mayo Radiography Program
Mayo Clinic/Foundation
Assistant Professor of Radiology
Mayo Medical School
Rochester, Minnesota

Sonya R. Lawson, M.S., R.T.(R) (T) (QM)
Assistant Professor and Clinical Coordinator
Department of Radiation Sciences
Virginia Commonwealth University/
  Medical College of Virginia Campus
Richmond, Virginia

Elizabeth L. Meixner, M.Ed., R.T.(R) (MR)
Assistant Chair
Department of Radiation Sciences
Virginia Commonwealth University/
  Medical College of Virginia Campus
Richmond, Virginia

Mary Jo Bergman, M.Ed., R.N., R.T.(R)
Program Director
Medcenter One Health Systems
Radiology Program
Bismarck, North Dakota

William J. Callaway, B.A., R.T.(R)
Director, Associate Degree Radiography
  Program
Chair, Allied Health Department
Lincoln Land Community College
Springfield, Illinois

Kimberley E. Krapels, R.T.(R)(M)
Instructor
Middlesex County College
Radiography Education Department
Edison, New Jersey

John T. Leesburg, M.A., R.T.(R)
Program Director
Jefferson State Community College
Birmingham, Alabama

James E. Mayhew, B.S., R.T.(R)
Clinical Coordinator
Ferris State University
Radiography Program
Big Rapids, Michigan

Linda Shields, M.Ed., R.T.
Instructor
Department of Health Occupations
El Paso Community College
El Paso, Texas

Diane Skog, R.T.(R)(T)
Clinical Data Coordinator
Oncology Administration
Maine Medical Center
Scarborough, Maine

O. Scott Staley, M.S., R.T.(R)
Assistant Professor
Radiologic Sciences Department
Boise State University
Boise, Idaho

James B. Temme, M.P.A., R.T.(R)
Program Director, Radiography
Associate Professor
University of Nebraska Medical Center
Omaha, Nebraska

Andrew P. Woodward,
  M.A., R.T.(R)(QM)(CT)(ARRT)
Radiologic Technology Department Head
Assistant Professor
WOR-WIC Community College
Salisbury, Maryland

Gary L. Watkins, Ph.D., R.T. (R)

1958–1998

This book is dedicated to the memory of Gary L. Watkins, Ph.D., R.T.(R), who died in July 1998. At the time of his death, Dr. Watkins was a tenured Associate Professor of Radiographic Science at Idaho State University in Pocatello. Before joining the faculty at Idaho State University in 1986, Dr. Watkins worked as a radiographer at Medical City Dallas Hospital in Dallas, Texas, and at the Good Samaritan Medical Center in Phoenix, Arizona.

Dr. Watkins earned his doctorate in adult education in 1996 after completing a master degree in educational technology in 1985. In his graduate and doctoral studies, Dr. Watkins focused on the art of instructional design, development, and evaluation, most particularly on the effect of CD-ROM and other media instruction on student achievement. His professional publications reflect a commitment both to the teaching and to the practice of radiography. It was Dr. Watkins's desire to better educate radiographers that motivated him to conceive of *Radiographic Imaging & Exposure* and to complete, with Dr. Terri Fauber, its first draft.

We are grateful for the clarity of vision and expression that Dr. Watkins provided, and we trust that the publication of this book honors his memory as a well-respected educator.

Radiographic Imaging & Exposure provides a fundamental presentation of topics that are important for students to master to be competent radiographers. Radiographers will also benefit from the practical approach to the topics of imaging and exposure presented here. Historically in the United States, the most common reason for repeat radiographic studies has been improper exposure, and radiographic exposure remains one of the most difficult subjects for student radiographers to master. Unfortunately, the proliferation of imaging and exposure textbooks in recent years has not been matched by an improved rate of producing quality radiographs. *Radiographic Imaging & Exposure* takes a unique and more effective approach to teaching the skills required by focusing on the practical fundamentals of imaging and exposure. With a topic such as radiographic imaging, it is impossible to depart from theoretic information entirely, and we do not want to. This book highlights the practical application of theoretic information to make it more immediately useful to students and practicing radiographers alike. Our ultimate goal is to provide the knowledge to problem solve effectively to consistently produce quality radiographic images in the clinical environment.

Content and Organization

Radiographic Imaging & Exposure begins with an intriguing discussion of Wilhelm Conrad Roentgen's discovery of x-rays in 1895 and the excitement it first caused among nineteenth-century society, who feared that private anatomy would be exposed for all to see! This introductory chapter moves into the realm of radiologic science with discussions of x-rays as energy and the unique characteristics of x-rays. Chapter 2 continues with a more detailed discussion of the x-ray beam, which is followed by chapters on radiographic image formation (Chapter 3), radiographic image quality (Chapter 4), scatter control (Chapter 5), and image receptors (Chapter 6). Chapter 7 is devoted to radiographic processing and includes important considerations regarding the darkroom environment and film handling. Chapter 8 provides a thorough discussion of sensitometry, including important clinical considerations. The next three chapters make up the exposure portion of *Radiographic Imaging & Exposure*: exposure factor selection (Chapter 9), automatic exposure control (Chapter 10), and exposure factor modification (Chapter 11). The final chapter is devoted to computed radiography, including fluoroscopy, to ensure that you understand the computer imaging process. This chapter explains the process of acquiring and displaying digital images and discusses the advantages and limitations of digital and conventional imaging processes.

Unique Features

Radiographic imaging and exposure is a complex topic, though a mastery of the fundamentals is necessary to become competent, whether you are a student or practicing radiographer. Three special features have been integrated within each chapter to facilitate the understanding and retention of the concepts under discussion and to underscore their applicability in a clinical setting. Each feature is distinguished by its own icon for easy recognition. The topic of radiographic imaging and exposure is replete with fundamental, important relationships, and they are emphasized in short,

meaningful ways at every opportunity. Important Relationships ▮ summarize the relationships being discussed in the text, as each one occurs, for immediate summary and review. Radiographic imaging also has a strong

quantitative component, and Mathematical Applications ▮ demonstrate the importance of mathematical formulas. This feature will help accustom you to the necessity of mastering mathematical formulas, and because they are presented with clinical scenarios, they provide immediate application

and explanation. Practical Tips ▮ also provide immediate application of the concepts under discussion by showing how they are applied in clinical practice. The information in the chapters thus comes to life and encourages you to actively imagine how you would apply the knowledge you are learning in the classroom in a clinical setting. These special features also give the practicing radiographer quick visual access to fundamental information that they need every day.

Learning Aids

One of the primary goals of *Radiographic Imaging & Exposure* is to be a practical textbook that will prepare student radiographers for the responsibilities of radiographic imaging in a clinical setting. Every effort has been made to make the material accessible and clear while remaining thorough. The writing style is straightforward and concise, and the textbook includes a number of features to aid in the mastery of its content. Relevant chapters

include Film Critique sections that provide the opportunity to apply the science of imaging and exposure to the art of assessing actual radiographic image quality. Interpretations of the images in the Film Critique sections are collected in a final appendix for reference and discussion. All of the Important Relationships, Mathematical Applications, and Practical Tips are also collected in three separate appendices for quick reference and review. These appendices are organized by chapter and include page references to the appearance of each entry in the text. *Radiographic Imaging & Exposure* includes the traditional learning aids as well. Each chapter begins with a list of objectives and key terms and concludes with a set of multiple-choice review questions, which will help you evaluate whether you have achieved the chapter's objectives. An answer key is provided in the back of the book.

Teaching Aids

An instructor's manual contains material that is useful for both the practiced and novice educator. Each chapter features a set of learning objectives, different from the objectives listed in the text and designed specifically for the instructor. These objectives pull out and organize the key concepts of the chapters. The teaching strategies then provide ideas for how to help your students really understand these concepts in addition to helping them master the stated chapter objectives. Usefulness is the key to the laboratory sections as well. The laboratories accommodate different resources and instructor preferences by including both examples of predesigned laboratory experiments and additional recommended laboratory activities. We are also pleased to include more than 100 transparency masters of line drawings, boxes, and tables from the textbook. Finally, to further help you in your classroom instruction, we have provided a test bank of 200 questions, divided by chapter.

Related Multimedia

Wherever appropriate, we have included links in the instructor's manual to *Mosby's Radiographic Instructional Series: Radiographic Imaging*. This multimedia tool provides an additional resource to help in the mastery of the topics in *Radiographic Imaging & Exposure*. Mosby has developed multimedia presentations of basic physics, imaging, radiobiology, and radiation protection. These presentations are available in both slide/audiotape and CD-ROM formats.

We hope that this book will help you prepare for a successful career in radiography and that it will continue to serve you well in your clinical practice.

Terri L. Fauber

ACKNOWLEDGMENTS

It takes many dedicated people to create a textbook that will add to the body of knowledge on radiographic imaging and exposure. This textbook is a compilation of the creative works of its contributors, along with the support and encouragement from Mosby editors. Jeanne Wilke, Carole Glauser, and Jennifer Genett have demonstrated great patience and persistence in supporting this project throughout its journey. In addition, the many reviewers were instrumental in ensuring the book's focus and integrity. The vision Gary Watkins provided during the initial stages of this project was truly the driving force behind a practical textbook for radiographic imaging. Last, radiography students' inquisitiveness and true desire for learning has inspired me to bridge the gap between radiographic imaging theory and practice.

Terri L. Fauber

CONTENTS

RADIATION AND ITS DISCOVERY *1*

THE X-RAY BEAM *12*

RADIOGRAPHIC IMAGE FORMATION *40*

RADIOGRAPHIC IMAGE QUALITY *50*

SCATTER CONTROL *100*

IMAGE RECEPTORS *134*

RADIOGRAPHIC PROCESSING *160*

SENSITOMETRY *192*

EXPOSURE FACTOR SELECTION *214*

AUTOMATIC EXPOSURE CONTROL *228*

EXPOSURE FACTOR MODIFICATION *248*

COMPUTED RADIOGRAPHY *268*

APPENDIX A SUMMARY OF IMPORTANT RELATIONSHIPS *290*

APPENDIX B SUMMARY OF MATHEMATICAL APPLICATIONS *304*

APPENDIX C SUMMARY OF PRACTICAL TIPS *310*

APPENDIX D FILM CRITIQUE INTERPRETATIONS *318*

ANSWER KEY *326*

CHAPTER 1

Radiation and Its Discovery

DISCOVERY

X-RAYS AS ENERGY

PROPERTIES OF X-RAYS

REVIEW QUESTIONS

1 Define all of the key terms in this chapter.

2 State all of the important relationships in this chapter.

3 Describe the events surrounding the discovery of x-rays.

4 Describe the dual nature of x-ray energy.

5 State the characteristics of electromagnetic radiation.

6 List the properties of x-rays.

fluorescence
electromagnetic radiation
wavelength

frequency
photon
quantum

X-rays were discovered in Europe in the late nineteenth century by German scientist Wilhelm Conrad Roentgen. Although Roentgen discovered x-rays by accident, he proceeded to study them so thoroughly that within a very short time, he had identified all of the properties of x-rays that are recognized today. Roentgen was less interested in the practical use of x-rays than in their characteristics as a form of energy. X-rays are classified as a specific type of energy termed *electromagnetic radiation*, but like all other types of electromagnetic energy, x-rays act both like waves and like particles.

Discovery

X-rays were discovered on November 8, 1895, by Dr. Wilhelm Conrad Roentgen (Figure 1-1), a German physicist and mathematician. Roentgen studied at the Polytechnic Institute in Zurich. He was appointed to the faculty of the University of

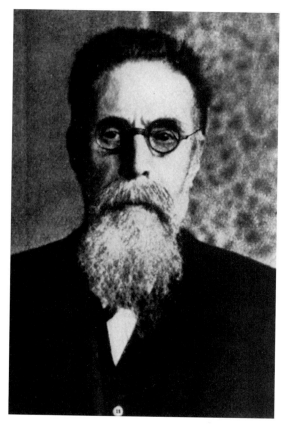

FIGURE 1-1 Dr. Wilhelm Conrad Roentgen. *From Glasser O:* Wilhelm Conrad Roentgen and the early history of the roentgen rays, *1933. Courtesy Charles C Thomas, Springfield, Ill.*

Würzburg and was their director of the Physical Institute at the time of his discovery. As a teacher and researcher, his academic interest dealt with the conduction of high-voltage electricity through low-vacuum tubes. A low-vacuum tube is simply a glass tube that has had some of the air evacuated from it. The specific type of tube that Roentgen was working with was called a *Crookes tube* (Figure 1-2).

Upon ending his work day on November 8, Roentgen prepared his research apparatus for the next experimental session to be conducted when he would return to his workplace. He darkened his laboratory to observe the electrical glow that occurred when the tube was energized. This glow from the tube would indicate that the tube was receiving electricity and ready to go for the next experiment. On this day, however, when Roentgen prepared his apparatus for the next experiment, as was his usual procedure, he noticed another faint glow, but this time it was external to his tube. This glow was coming from some material located about 1 m from his electrified tube. Astonished, Roentgen covered his tube with opaque black paper and again electrified the tube to ascertain the precise source of this faint glow. The source was a piece of paper coated with barium platinocyanide. Each time Roentgen energized his tube, he observed this glow coming from the barium platinocyanide paper. He understood that energy emanating from his tube was causing this paper to produce light, or fluoresce. **Fluorescence** refers to the instantaneous production of light resulting from the interaction of some type of energy (in this case x-rays) and some element or compound (in this case barium platinocyanide).

Roentgen was understandably excited about this apparent discovery, but he was also cautious not to make any early assumptions about what he had observed. Before sharing information about his discovery with colleagues, Roentgen spent time meticulously investigating the properties of this new type of energy. Of course, this new type of energy was not new at all. It had always existed and was likely produced by Roentgen and his contemporaries who were also involved in experiments with

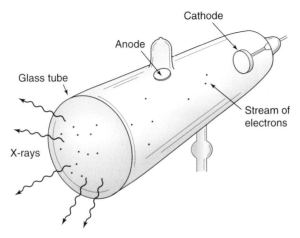

FIGURE 1-2 A Crookes tube as used by Roentgen to discover x-rays.

electricity and low-vacuum tubes. Knowing that others were doing similar research, Roentgen worked in earnest to determine just what this energy was.

Roentgen spent the next several weeks working feverishly in his laboratory to investigate as many properties of this energy as he could. He noticed that when he placed his hand between his energized tube and the barium platinocyanide–coated paper, he could see the bones of his hand glow on the paper with this fluoroscopic image moving as he moved his hand. Curious about this, he produced a static image of his wife Anna Bertha's hand using a 15-minute exposure. This became the world's first radiograph (Figure 1-3). Roentgen then gathered other materials and interposed them between his energized tube and the fluorescent paper. Some materials, such as wood, allowed this energy to pass through it and caused the paper to fluoresce. Some, such as platinum, did not.

In December 1895, Roentgen decided that his investigations of this energy were complete enough that it was time to inform his physicist colleagues of what he now believed to indeed be a discovery of a new form of energy. He called this energy x-rays with the *x* representing the mathematical symbol of the unknown. On

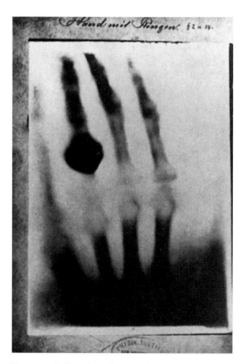

FIGURE 1-3 The first radiograph, that of Roentgen's wife, Anna Bertha, demonstrating the bones of her hand with a ring on one finger. *From Glasser O: Wilhelm Conrad Roentgen and the early history of the roentgen rays, 1933. Courtesy Charles C Thomas, Springfield, Ill.*

December 28, 1895, Roentgen submitted a scholarly paper on his research activities to his local professional society, the Würzburg Physico-Medical Society. Written in his native German, his article was titled "On a new kind of rays," and it caused a buzz of excitement in the medical and scientific communities. Fairly quickly, an English translation of this article appeared in the journal *Nature*, dated January 23, 1896.

Roentgen viewed his discovery as an important one to be certain, but he also viewed it as one of primarily academic interest. His interest was in the x-ray itself as a form of energy, not in the possible practical uses of it. Others quickly began assembling their own x-ray–producing devices and exposed inanimate objects as well as tissue, both animal and human, both living and dead, to determine the range of use of these x-rays. Their efforts were driven largely on the basis of skepticism, not believing that x-rays could do what they had believed had been claimed. Skepticism eventually gave way to productive curiosity as investigations concentrated on ways of imaging the living human body for medical benefit.

As investigations into legitimate medical applications of the use of x-rays continued, the nonmedical and nonscientific communities were taking a different view of Roentgen's discovery. X-ray–proof underwear was offered as protection from these rays that were known to penetrate solid materials. A New Jersey legislator attempted to enact legislation that would ban the use of x-ray–producing devices in opera glasses. Both of these efforts were presumably aimed at protecting one from revealing their private anatomy to the unscrupulous users of x-rays. The public furor reached such a height that a London newspaper, the *Pall Mall Gazette*, offered the following editorial in 1896: "We are sick of Roentgen rays. Perhaps the best thing would be for all civilized nations to combine to burn all the Roentgen rays, to execute all the discoverers, and to corner all the equipment in the world and to whelm it in the middle of the ocean. Let the fish contemplate each other's bones if they like, but not us."

In a similar vein, but in a more creative fashion, another London newspaper, *Photography*, in 1896 offered the following:

> Roentgen Rays, Roentgen Rays?
> What is this craze?
> The town's ablaze
> With this new phase
> Of x-ray ways.
> I'm full of daze, shock and amaze,
> For nowadays
> I hear they'll gaze
> Through cloak and gown and even stays!
> The naughty, naughty Roentgen rays!"

Fortunately for the benefit of society, the scientific applications of x-rays continued to be investigated, despite these public distractions. Roentgen's discovery was indeed lauded as one of great significance to science and medicine. Roentgen received the first-ever Nobel prize for physics in 1901. The branch of medicine that was concerned with using x-rays was called *roentgenology*. A unit of radiation exposure was called the *roentgen*. X-rays were, for a time at least, called *roentgen rays*.

Excitement over this previously undiscovered type of energy was somewhat tempered by the realization in 1898 that x-rays could cause biologic damage. This was first noticed as a reddening and burning of the skin of those who were exposed to the large doses of x-rays required at that time. More serious effects, such as the growth of malignant tumors and the alteration of one's chromosomes, were attributed in later decades to x-ray exposure. Despite these disturbing findings, however, it was also realized that x-rays could be used safely. When radiation-protection behaviors that protect both radiographer and patient are used, x-rays are useful in imaging virtually every part of the human body for the purpose of medical diagnosis.

X-Rays as Energy

X-radiation, or x-rays, are a type of electromagnetic radiation. **Electromagnetic radiation** refers to radiation that has both electrical and magnetic properties. All radiations that are electromagnetic comprise a spectrum (Figure 1-4).

In the academic discipline of physics, energy can generally be described as behaving according to the wave concept of physics or the particle concept of physics. X-rays have a dual nature in that they behave both like waves and like particles.

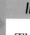

Important Relationship

The Dual Nature of X-Ray Energy

X-rays act both like waves and like particles.

X-rays can be described as waves because they move in waves that have wavelength and frequency. If a sine wave were to be observed (Figure 1-5), it would be seen that **wavelength** represents the distance between two successive crests or troughs. Wavelength is represented by the Greek letter lambda (λ), and values are given in units of angstroms (Å). X-rays used in radiography range in wavelength from about 0.1 to 1.0 Å.

The sine wave (see Figure 1-5) also demonstrates that **frequency** represents the number of waves passing a given point per given unit of time. Frequency is represented by a lowercase *f* or by the Greek letter nu (ν), and values are given in units of Hertz (Hz). X-rays used in radiography range in frequency from about 3×10^{19} to 3×10^{18} Hz. Wavelength and frequency are inversely related. That is, as one increases, the other decreases, and as one decreases, the other increases.

THE ELECTROMAGNETIC SPECTRUM

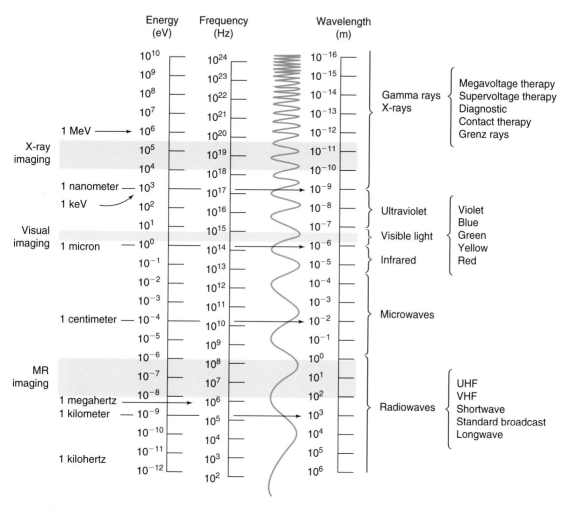

FIGURE 1-4 The electromagnetic spectrum. Radiowaves are the least energetic on the spectrum, and gamma rays are the most energetic.

Important Relationship

Wavelength and Frequency

Wavelength and frequency are inversely related. If one increases, the other decreases.

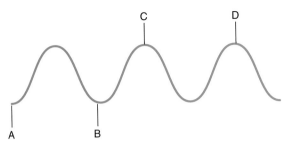

FIGURE 1-5 A sine wave demonstrating wavelength and frequency. One wavelength is equal to the distance between two successive troughs (points *A* to *B*) or the distance between two successive crests (points *C* to *D*).

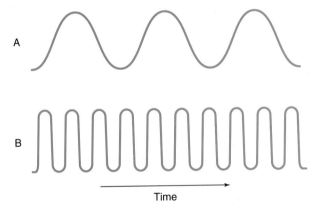

FIGURE 1-6 Sine wave **A** demonstrates long wavelength and low frequency. Sine wave **B** demonstrates short wavelength and high frequency. A comparison of sine waves **A** and **B** demonstrates the inverse relationship of wavelength and frequency.

This relationship can be observed in Figure 1-6 and is demonstrated by the expression $c = \lambda \nu$, where *c* represents the speed of light. In this expression, if wavelength increases, frequency must decrease because the speed of light is a constant velocity (3×10^8 m/s, or 186,000 miles/s). Conversely, if wavelength decreases, frequency must increase, again because the speed of light is constant.

X-rays also behave like particles and move as photons or quanta (plural). A **photon** or **quantum** (singular) is a small, discrete bundle of energy. For most applications in radiography, x-rays are referred to as *photons*. The energy of an individual photon is measured in units of electron volts (eV) and can be indicated by one of three expressions:

$$E = h\nu, \text{ or } E = hc/\lambda, \text{ or } E = 12.4/\lambda$$

where

E = Photon energy
h = Planck's constant (6.62×10^{-34} joules seconds)
c = The speed of light
ν = Frequency
λ = Wavelength.

Properties of X-Rays

X-rays are known to have several characteristics or properties. These characteristics are briefly explained here and presented in Box 1-1.

- *X-rays are invisible.* In addition to not being able to see x-rays, one can also not feel, smell, or hear them.
- *X-rays are electrically neutral.* They have neither a positive nor a negative charge; therefore they cannot be accelerated or made to change direction by a magnet or electrical field.
- *X-rays have no mass.* They create no resistance to being put into motion and cannot produce force.
- *X-rays travel at the speed of light in a vacuum.* They move at a constant velocity of 3×10^8 m/s or 186,000 miles/s in a vacuum.

Box 1-1 *Characteristics of X-Rays*

Are invisible.
Are electrically neutral.
Have no mass.
Travel at the speed of light in a vacuum.
Cannot be optically focused.
Form a polyenergetic or heterogenous beam.
Can be produced in a range of energies.
Travel in straight lines.
Can cause some substances to fluoresce.
Cause chemical changes in radiographic and photographic film.
Can penetrate the human body.
Can be absorbed or scattered in the human body.
Can produce secondary radiation.
Can cause damage to living tissue.

- *X-rays cannot be optically focused.* Optical lenses have no ability in focusing or refracting x-ray photons.

- *X-rays form a polyenergetic or heterogenous beam.* The x-ray beam that is used in diagnostic radiography comprises many photons that have many different energies. The maximum energy that a photon in any beam may have is expressed by the kilovoltage peak (kVp) that is set on the control panel of the radiographic unit by the radiographer.

- *X-rays can be produced in a range of energies.* These are useful for different purposes in diagnostic radiography. The medically useful range of x-ray energies extends from 20 to 150 kVp.

- *X-rays travel in straight lines.* X-rays used in diagnostic radiography form a divergent beam in which each individual photon travels in a straight line.

- *X-rays can cause some substances to fluoresce.* When x-rays strike some substances, those substances produce light. These substances are used to advantage in diagnostic radiography in intensifying screens and in image intensifiers used in fluoroscopy.

- *X-rays cause chemical changes to occur in radiographic and photographic film.* X-rays are capable of causing images to appear on radiographic film and are capable of fogging photographic film.

- *X-rays can penetrate the human body.* X-rays have the ability to pass through the body, based on the energy of the x-rays and on the composition and thickness of the tissues being exposed.

- *X-rays can be absorbed or scattered by tissues in the human body.* Depending on the energy of an individual x-ray photon, that photon may be absorbed in the body or be made to scatter, moving in another direction.

- *X-rays can produce secondary radiation.* When x-rays are absorbed as a result of a specific type of interaction with matter, the photoelectric effect, a secondary or characteristic photon will be produced.

- *X-rays can cause chemical and biologic damage to living tissue.* Through excitation and ionization of atoms comprising cells, damage to those cells can occur.

Since the publication of Roentgen's scientific paper, no other properties of x-rays have been discovered. However, the discussion of x-rays has expanded far beyond the early concerns about modesty or even danger. Today, x-rays are accepted as an important diagnostic tool in medicine, and the radiographer is an important member of the health care team. The radiographic imaging professional is responsible for the care of the patient in the radiology department, as well as for the production and control of x-rays and the formation of the radiographic image. The balance of this book uncovers the intricate and fascinating details of the art and science of medical radiography.

Review Questions

1. In what year were x-rays discovered?
   A. 1892
   B. 1895
   C. 1898
   D. 1901

2. In what year were some of the biologically damaging effects of x-rays discovered?
   A. 1892
   B. 1895
   C. 1898
   D. 1901

3. X-rays were discovered in experiments dealing with electricity and
   A. ionization.
   B. magnetism.
   C. atomic structure.
   D. vacuum tubes.

4. X-rays were discovered when they caused a barium platinocyanide plate to
   A. fluoresce.
   B. phosphoresce.
   C. vibrate.
   D. burn and redden.

5. X-radiation is part of the _____ spectrum.
   A. radiation
   B. energy
   C. atomic
   D. electromagnetic

6. X-rays have a dual nature, which means that they behave like both
   A. atoms and molecules.
   B. photons and quanta.
   C. waves and particles.
   D. charged and uncharged particles.

7. The wavelength and frequency of x-rays are _____ related.
   A. directly
   B. inversely
   C. partially
   D. not

8. X-rays have a(n) _____ electrical charge.
   A. positive
   B. negative
   C. alternately positive and negative
   D. no charge

9. X-rays have
   A. no mass.
   B. the same mass as electrons.
   C. the same mass as protons.
   D. the same mass as neutrons.

10. The x-ray beam used in diagnostic radiography can be described as being
    A. homogenous.
    B. monoenergetic.
    C. polyenergetic.
    D. scattered.

CHAPTER 2

The X-Ray Beam

X-RAY PRODUCTION

Cathode
Anode
X-Ray Tube Housing
Recent Innovations

TARGET INTERACTIONS

Bremsstrahlung Interactions
Characteristic Interactions

X-RAY EMISSION SPECTRUM

X-RAY EXPOSURE

X-RAY QUALITY AND QUANTITY

Kilovoltage
Milliamperage
Exposure Time
Milliamperage and Time

LINE FOCUS PRINCIPLE

ANODE HEEL EFFECT

BEAM FILTRATION

Half-Value Layer
Special Filters

HEAT UNITS

TUBE RATING CHARTS

EXTENDING X-RAY TUBE LIFE

REVIEW QUESTIONS

1 Define all of the key terms in this chapter.

2 State all of the important relationships in this chapter.

3 Describe construction of the x-ray tube.

4 State the function of each component of the x-ray tube.

5 Describe how x-rays are produced.

6 Explain the role of the primary exposure factors in determining the quality and quantity of x-rays.

7 Explain the line focus principle.

8 State how the anode heel effect can be used in radiography.

9 State the purpose of an instantaneous load tube rating chart.

10 List the guidelines followed to extend the life of an x-ray tube.

KEY TERMS

cathode
filament
focusing cup
anode
target
stator
rotor
focal spot
leakage radiation
bremsstrahlung interactions
characteristic interactions
x-ray emission spectrum
filament current
thermionic emission
space charge

space charge effect
tube current
line focus principle
actual focal spot size
effective focal spot size
anode heel effect
added filtration
inherent filtration
total filtration
half-value layer (HVL)
compensating filter
wedge filter
trough filter
heat unit (HU)
instantaneous load tube rating chart

The x-ray tube is the most important part of the x-ray machine because the tube is where the x-rays are actually produced. Radiographers must understand how the x-ray tube is constructed and how to operate it. The radiographer controls many of the actions that occur within the tube. Kilovoltage peak (kVp), milliamperage (mA), exposure time, and milliampere seconds (mAs) are all factors that the radiographer selects to produce a quality image. The radiographer also needs to be aware of the amount of heat that is produced during x-ray production because excessive heat can damage the tube.

X-Ray Production

The production of x-rays requires a rapidly moving stream of electrons that are suddenly decelerated or stopped. The source of electrons is the cathode, or negative electrode. Electrons are stopped or decelerated by the anode, or positive electrode. Electrons move between the cathode and the anode because there is a potential difference in charge between the electrodes.

CATHODE

The **cathode** of an x-ray tube is a negatively charged electrode. It comprises a filament and a focusing cup. Figure 2-1 demonstrates a double-filament cathode surrounded by a focusing cup. The **filament** is a coiled tungsten wire that serves as the source of electrons during x-ray production.

Important Relationship

The Filament

The filament is the source of electrons during x-ray production.

Most x-ray tubes are referred to as *dual-focus tubes* because they use two filaments: a large filament and a small filament. Only one filament is energized at any one time during x-ray production. If the radiographer chooses a large focal spot, the large filament is energized. If a small focal spot is chosen, the small filament is energized.

The **focusing cup** is made of nickel and mostly surrounds the filament. It is open at one end to allow electrons to flow freely across the tube from cathode to anode. Its purpose is to focus the stream of electrons before they strike the anode.

Important Relationship

Focusing the Electron Stream

The negatively charged focusing cup condenses the stream of electrons flowing from the cathode and focuses, or directs, it to the anode.

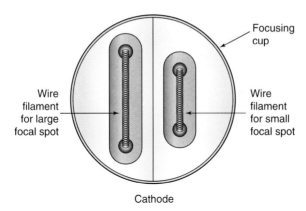

FIGURE 2-1 Most x-ray tubes use a small filament and a large filament, corresponding with a small focal spot size and a large focal spot size.

ANODE

The **anode** of an x-ray tube is a positively charged electrode. It consists of a target and, in rotating anode tubes, a stator and rotor. The **target** is a metal that abruptly decelerates and stops electrons in the tube current, thereby allowing for the production of x-rays. The target can be either rotating or stationary. Rotating target tubes are more common than stationary ones. Rotating anodes are manufactured to rotate at a set speed ranging from 3000 to 10,000 revolutions per minute (RPM). Figure 2-2 demonstrates the difference in the appearance of a rotating and stationary target.

Important Relationship

The Target

The target is the part of the anode that is struck by the focused stream of electrons coming from the cathode. The target stops the electrons and thus creates the opportunity of the production of x-rays.

The target of rotating anode tubes is made of a tungsten and rhenium alloy. This layer, or track, is then embedded in a base of molybdenum and graphite (Figure 2-3). Tungsten generally makes up 90% of the composition of the rotating target, with rhenium making up the other 10%. Rotating targets generally have a target angle ranging from 6 to 20 degrees. Tungsten is used in both rotating and stationary targets because it has a high atomic number of 74 for efficient x-ray production and because it has a high melting point of 3370° F. Most of the energy produced by an x-ray tube is heat, so melting of the target can sometimes become a problem, especially at high exposure factors.

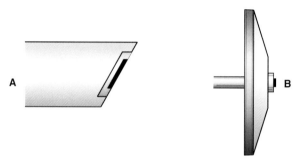

FIGURE 2-2 Side views of (**A**) a stationary anode and (**B**) a rotating anode.

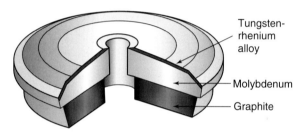

Tungsten-rhenium alloy

Molybdenum

Graphite

FIGURE 2-3 Typical construction of a rotating anode.

Important Relationship

Tungsten

Because tungsten has a high atomic number (74) and a high melting point (3370° F), it efficiently produces x-rays.

Almost all x-ray tube targets are made of tungsten. The only exception is the target of mammography x-ray machines. In mammography machines, molybdenum comprises 97% of the target. Like tungsten, molybdenum has a high melting point, but unlike tungsten, it produces a much lower-energy x-ray beam. An x-ray beam with lower energy is necessary for breast imaging so that the breast tissue can be better differentiated.

The **stator** is an electric motor that rotates the rotor at very high speed during x-ray production. The **rotor** is rigidly connected to the target through the anode stem, causing the target to rotate rapidly during x-ray production. Very-high-strength bearings in the rotor allow it to rotate smoothly at high speeds.

The purpose of the anode is also to dissipate heat away from the tube so that the tube is not damaged. Heat is transferred from the target through the anode stem

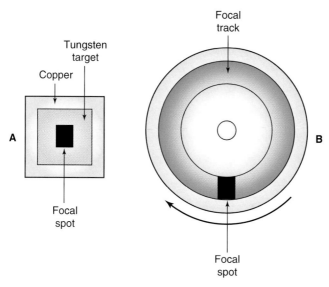

FIGURE 2-4 A, Front view of a rotating anode. **B,** The target area of the rotating anode turns during exposure, and there is an increased physical area, a focal track, that is exposed to electrons.

and to the rotor. The heat is then transferred to the glass envelope and to the insulating oil that surrounds the x-ray tube. Many tube assemblies also have a fan to blow air over the tube to help dissipate heat.

Important Relationship

Dissipating Heat

As the target rotates and heat within the tube increases, the anode conducts heat to the insulating oil that surrounds the x-ray tube.

Rotating anodes can withstand large heat loads. The ability to withstand high heat loads has to do, in part, with the **focal spot,** which is the physical area of the target that is exposed to electrons during x-ray production. With stationary targets the focal spot is a fixed area on the surface of the target. With rotating targets this area is represented by a focal track. Figure 2-4 shows the rotating anode and its focal track. The size of the focal spot does not change with a rotating target, but the actual physical area of the target that is exposed to electrons is constantly rotating, causing a greater physical area, a focal track, to be exposed to electrons. Because of the larger physical target area, the rotating target is able to withstand larger heat loads produced by greater exposure factors. Rotating anode x-ray tubes are used in all applications in radiography.

Important Relationship

Rotating Anodes

Rotating anodes can withstand greater heat loads than stationary anodes because their rotating motion causes a greater physical area, or focal track, to be exposed to electrons.

X-RAY TUBE HOUSING

The components necessary for x-ray production are housed in a glass envelope. Figure 2-5 illustrates the structure of an x-ray tube, and Figure 2-6 shows the appearance of a typical x-ray tube. The glass envelope allows air to be evacuated completely from the x-ray tube, allowing the efficient flow of electrons across the tube gap from cathode to anode. The glass envelope serves two additional functions: it provides some insulation from electrical shock that may occur because the cathode and anode contain electrical charges, and it dissipates heat in the tube by conducting it to the insulating oil that surrounds the glass envelope. The purpose of insulating oil is to provide more insulation from electrical shock and also to help dissipate heat away from the tube. All of these components are surrounded by a metal tube housing. It is the metal tube housing that the radiographer actually sees and handles when moving the x-ray tube. The tube housing is lined with lead to provide some shielding from leakage radiation. **Leakage radiation** refers to any x-rays that escape the tube housing. The tube housing is required to allow no more than 100 mR/hr of leakage radiation to escape when measured at 1 m from the source while the tube operates at maximum output. Electrical current is supplied to the x-ray tube by means of two high-voltage cables that enter the top of the tube assembly.

RECENT INNOVATIONS

Two recent innovations in the design of modern diagnostic x-ray tubes have made them more efficient. One of these is the metal center section x-ray tube. A metal center section replaces the glass envelope in this region. In traditional x-ray tubes, tungsten that is evaporated from the filament during exposure deposits on the inside of the glass envelope, especially in the center of this envelope. This evaporation decreases the insulating ability of the tube and could lead to breakage of the glass, causing the tube to fail. Replacing this section of glass with metal prevents these problems and extends the tube life. The other innovation is the bonding of graphite to the back of the molybdenum disk used

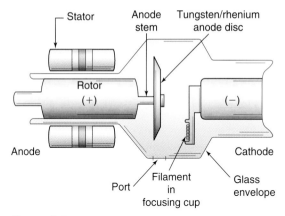

FIGURE 2-5 Structure of a typical x-ray tube, including the major operational parts.

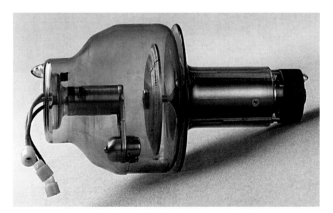

FIGURE 2-6 A typical x-ray tube as it appears before installation in a tube housing.

in rotating targets. Graphite has a high melting temperature and greatly assists in dissipating heat away from the tube.

Target Interactions

The electrons that move from the cathode to the anode travel extremely fast, approximately half the speed of light. The moving electrons, having kinetic energy, strike the target and interact with the tungsten atoms in the anode to produce x-rays.

Important Relationship

The Production of X-Rays

As electrons strike the target, their kinetic energy is transferred to the tungsten atoms in the anode to produce x-rays.

These interactions occur within the top 0.5 mm of the anode surface. Two types of interaction produce x-ray photons: bremsstrahlung interactions and characteristic interactions.

Important Relationship

Interactions That Produce X-Ray Photons

Bremsstrahlung interactions and characteristic interactions both produce x-ray photons.

BREMSSTRAHLUNG INTERACTIONS

Bremsstrahlung is a German word meaning "braking" or "slowing down." **Bremsstrahlung interactions** occur when a projectile electron completely avoids the orbital electrons of the tungsten atom and travels very close to its nucleus. The very strong electrostatic force of the nucleus causes the electron to suddenly "slow down." As the electron looses energy, it suddenly changes its direction and the energy loss then reappears as an x-ray photon (Figure 2-7).

In the diagnostic energy range, most x-ray interactions are bremsstrahlung. The diagnostic energy range is 30 to 150 kVp. Below 70 kVp, 100% of the x-ray beam consists of bremsstrahlung interactions. Above 70 kVp, approximately 85% of the beam consists of bremsstrahlung interactions.

Important Relationship

Bremsstrahlung Interactions

Most x-ray interactions in the diagnostic energy range are bremsstrahlung.

CHARACTERISTIC INTERACTIONS

Characteristic interactions are produced when a projectile electron interacts with an electron from the inner K-shell of the tungsten atom. The electron must have enough energy to eject the K-shell electron from its orbit. When the K-shell

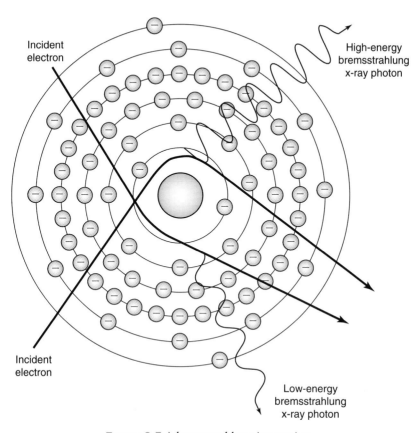

Incident
electron

High-energy
bremsstrahlung
x-ray photon

Incident
electron

Low-energy
bremsstrahlung
x-ray photon

FIGURE 2-7 A bremsstrahlung interaction.

electron is ejected from its orbit, an outer-shell electron drops into the open position and thereby creates an energy difference. The energy difference is emitted as
an x-ray photon (Figure 2-8). Electrons from the L-, M-, O-, and P-shells of the
tungsten atom are also ejected from their orbits. However, the photons created from
these interactions have very low energy and, depending on filtration, may not even
reach the patient. K-characteristic x-rays have an average energy of approximately
69 keV; therefore they contribute significantly to the useful x-ray beam. Below
70 kVp, no characteristic x-rays are present in the beam. Above 70 kVp, approximately 15% of the beam consists of characteristic x-rays. X-rays produced through
these interactions are termed *characteristic* x-rays because their energies are characteristic of the tungsten target element.

To summarize, when bremsstrahlung and characteristic interactions are compared, the great majority of x-ray interactions produced in diagnostic radiology are
produced by bremsstrahlung. There is no difference between a bremsstrahlung x-ray
and a characteristic x-ray at the same energy level; they are just produced by different processes.

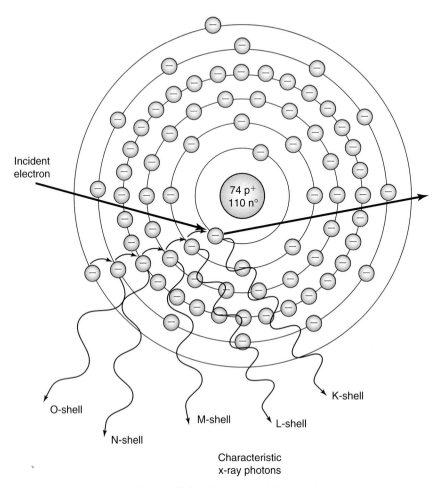

Incident
electron

74 p$^+$
110 n$^\circ$

O-shell

N-shell

M-shell

L-shell

K-shell

Characteristic
x-ray photons

FIGURE 2-8 A characteristic interaction.

X-Ray Emission Spectrum

X-ray energy is measured in kiloelectron-volts (keV) (1000 electron volts). The x-ray beam is polyenergenic and consists of a wide range of energies known as **x-ray emission spectrum.** The lowest energies will always be approximately 15 to 20 keV, and the highest energies will always be equal to the kVp set on the control panel. For example, an 80-kVp x-ray exposure technique will produce x-ray energies ranging from a low of 15 keV to a high of 80 keV (Figure 2-9). The fewest number of x-rays occurs at the extreme low and high ends of the spectrum. The greatest number of x-ray energies will occur between 30 and 40 keV for an 80-kVp exposure. The x-ray emission spectrum, or the range and intensity of x-rays emitted, will change with different exposure and kVp settings on the control panel.

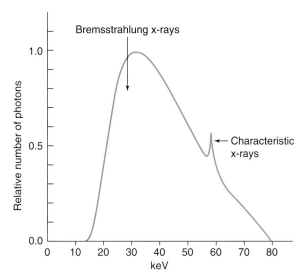

FIGURE 2-9 An 80-kVp x-ray emission spectrum from a tungsten target. Most x-rays occur between 30 and 40 keV.

X-Ray Exposure

A radiographic exposure is produced by a radiographer using two switches. These are sometimes combined into a single switching device that has two levels of operation corresponding with the first and second switches usually found on x-ray control panels. In either case the switches that are used to make an x-ray exposure are considered *deadman switches*. Deadman switches require positive pressure to be applied during the entire x-ray exposure process. If the radiographer lets off of either switch, releasing positive pressure, the exposure process is immediately terminated.

The first switch is usually called the *rotor*, or *prep*, *button*, and the second switch is usually called the *exposure*, or *x-ray*, *button*. The activation of each switch by the radiographer causes specific things to occur inside the x-ray tube. The rotor, or prep, button must be activated before the exposure, or x-ray, button is activated to properly produce an x-ray exposure.

Pushing the rotor, or prep, button causes a **filament current** to be induced across the filament. This filament current is relatively low, about 3 to 5 amp and operates at about 10 V. The filament current heats the tungsten filament. This heating of the filament causes thermionic emission to occur. **Thermionic emission** refers to the boiling off of electrons from the filament.

Important Relationship

Thermionic Emission

When the tungsten filament gains enough heat *(therm)*, the outer-shell electrons *(ions)* of the filament atoms are boiled off, or *emitted*, from the filament.

The electrons liberated from the filament during thermionic emission form a cloud around the filament called the **space charge.** This term is descriptive because there is an actual negative charge from these electrons that exists in space around the filament. **Space charge effect** refers to the tendency of the space charge to not allow more electrons to be boiled off of the filament.

By pushing the rotor, or prep, button, the radiographer also activates the stator that drives the rotor and rotating target (Box 2-1). While thermionic emission is occurring and the space charge is forming, the stator is starting to turn the anode, accelerating it to top speed in preparation for x-ray production. If an exposure could be made before the target is up to speed, the heat produced would be too great for the slowly rotating target, causing serious damage. The machine will not allow the exposure to take place until the target is up to full speed, even if the exposure switch is activated. Therefore the radiographer can press the rotor and exposure switches one right after the other, and the machine will make the exposure as soon as it is ready with no damage to the tube. It takes only a few seconds for the space charge to be produced and for the rotating target to reach its top speed (Figure 2-10). Usually, an audible click or other sound alerts the radiographer that the tube is ready to produce x-rays.

Box 2-1   *Preparing the Tube for Exposure*

When the rotor, or prep, button is pushed:

On the cathode side of the x-ray tube
1. Filament current heats up the filament.
2. This heat boils electrons off the filament (thermionic emission).
3. These electrons gather in a cloud around the filament (space charge).
4. The number of electrons in the space charge is limited (space charge effect).

On the anode side of the x-ray tube
1. The rotating target begins to turn rapidly, quickly reaching top speed.

When the radiographer pushes the exposure, or x-ray, button, the x-ray exposure begins (Box 2-2). The kVp level, depending on the actual kVp value set by the radiographer, is applied across the tube from cathode to anode. The cathode becomes highly negatively charged, strongly repelling the also negatively charged electrons away from it. The anode becomes positively charged, strongly attracting the electrons to it. Electrons that comprised the space charge now flow quickly from cathode to anode in a current. **Tube current** refers to the flow of electrons from cathode to anode and is measured in units called milliamperes (mA). It is important to note that electrons flow in only one direction in the x-ray tube—from cathode to anode.

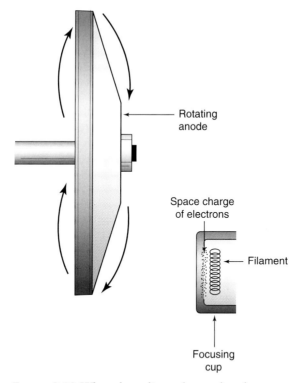

FIGURE 2-10 When the radiographer pushes the rotor, or prep, button, a filament current is induced across the filament, causing electrons to be burned off and gather in a cloud around the filament. At the same time, the rotating anode begins to turn.

When the exposure, or x-ray, button is pushed:

On the cathode side of the x-ray tube	On the anode side of the x-ray tube
1. High negative charge strongly repels electrons.	**1.** High positive charge strongly attracts electrons in the tube current.
2. These electrons stream away from the cathode and toward the anode (tube current).	**2.** These electrons strike the anode.
	3. X-rays and heat are produced.

Important Relationship

Tube Current

Electrons flow in only one direction in the x-ray tube—from cathode to anode. This flow of electrons is called the *tube current* and is measured in milliamperes (mA).

As these electrons strike the anode target, they are converted to either x-rays or heat. In other words, an energy conversion occurs. The kinetic energy of the moving electrons is changed to electromagnetic energy (x-rays) and thermal energy (heat). Most of the electrons in the tube current (approximately 99%) are converted to heat, whereas only approximately 1% of these electrons are converted to x-rays. These events are illustrated in Figure 2-11.

Important Relationship

Energy Conversion in the X-Ray Tube

As electrons strike the anode target, approximately 99% of their kinetic energy is converted to heat, whereas only approximately 1% is converted to x-rays.

X-Ray Quality and Quantity

The radiographer initiates and controls the production of x-rays. Manipulating the prime exposure factors on the control panel (kVp, mA, and exposure time) allows both the quantity and quality of the x-ray beam to be altered. The quantity of the x-ray beam indicates the number of x-ray photons in the primary beam, and the

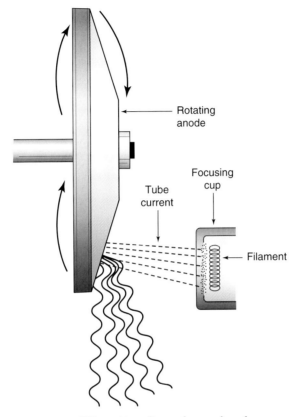

FIGURE 2-11 When the radiographer pushes the exposure, or x-ray, button, a high negative kilovoltage is induced across the cathode and a high positive kilovoltage is induced across the anode. Electrons are repelled from the cathode side and attracted to the anode side. The negatively charged focusing cup focuses the electrons into a stream, and they quickly cross the tube gap in a tube current. Electrons interacting with the target are converted into x-rays and heat.

quality of the x-ray beam indicates its penetrating power. Knowledge of the prime exposure factors and their effect on the production of x-rays will assist the radiographer in producing quality radiographs.

KILOVOLTAGE

The kilovoltage (kVp) that is set by the radiographer and applied across the x-ray tube at the time the exposure is initiated determines the speed at which the electrons in the tube current move.

Important Relationship

Kilovoltage and the Speed of Electrons

The speed of the electrons traveling from the cathode to the anode increases as the kilovoltage applied across the x-ray tube increases.

A higher voltage results in greater repulsion of electrons from the cathode and greater attraction of electrons toward the anode. The speed at which the electrons in the tube current move determines the quality or energy of the x-rays that are produced. When one refers to the x-ray photons themselves or to the primary beam, *quality* and *energy* mean the same thing (Box 2-3).

Important Relationship

The Speed of Electrons and the Quality of the X-Rays

The speed of the electrons in the tube current determines the quality or energy of the x-rays that are produced. The quality or energy of the x-rays that are produced determines the penetrability of the primary beam.

BOX 2-3 *kVp and X-Ray Quality*

1. Higher kVp results in electrons that move faster in the tube current from cathode to anode.
2. The faster the electrons in the tube current move, the greater the quality of the x-rays produced.
3. The greater the quality of the x-rays that are produced, the greater the penetrability of the primary beam.

Important Relationship

kVp and Beam Penetrability

As kVp increases, beam penetrability increases; as kVp decreases, beam penetrability decreases.

In addition to kVp having an effect on the quality of x-ray photons produced, kVp has an effect on the quantity or number of x-ray photons produced. Increased kVp results in more x-rays being produced because increased kVp increases the efficiency of x-ray production.

MILLIAMPERAGE

A milliampere (mA) is the unit used to measure the tube current. Tube current measures the number of electrons flowing per unit time between the cathode and anode. For example, 100 mA indicates the number of electrons flowing in the tube per second. Selecting the 200-mA station causes twice as many electrons to flow per second. The milliamperage that is set by the radiographer determines the number of electrons flowing in the tube and the quantity of x-rays produced (Box 2-4). The quantity of electrons in the tube current is directly proportional to the milliamperage. If the milliamperage increases, the quantity of electrons and the quantity of x-rays increases proportionally. If the milliamperage decreases, the quantity of electrons and the quantity of x-rays decreases by the same proportion. Milliamperage does not affect the quality of the x-rays produced.

Important Relationship

Milliamperage, Tube Current, and X-Ray Quantity

The quantity of electrons in the tube current and quantity of x-rays produced are directly proportional to the milliamperage.

Box 2-4 *mA and X-Ray Quantity*

1. Higher mA results in more electrons that move in the tube current from cathode to anode.
2. The more electrons in the tube current, the more x-rays that will be produced.
3. The number of x-rays that are produced is directly proportionate to the mA.

EXPOSURE TIME

Exposure time determines the length of time that the x-ray tube produces x-rays. The exposure time that is set by the radiographer can be expressed in seconds or milliseconds, either as a fraction or a decimal. This exposure time determines the length of time that the tube current is allowed to flow from cathode to anode. The longer the exposure time, the greater the quantity of electrons that will flow from the cathode to the anode and the greater the quantity of x-rays produced (Box 2-5). For example, if 400 mA at an exposure time of 0.25 second produces 100 x-rays, then an exposure time of 0.50 second at 400 mA will produce 200 x-rays. Changes in exposure time produce the same effect on the number of x-rays produced, as do changes in milliamperage.

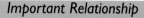

Important Relationship

Exposure Time, Tube Current, and X-Ray Quantity

The quantity of electrons that flows from cathode to anode and the quantity of x-rays produced are directly proportionate to the exposure time.

BOX 2-5 *Exposure Time and X-Ray Quantity*

1. Longer exposure time results in more electrons that move in the tube current from cathode to anode.
2. The more electrons in the tube current, the more x-rays produced.
3. The number of x-rays that are produced is directly proportionate to the exposure time.

MILLIAMPERAGE AND TIME

When milliamperage is multiplied by exposure time, the result is known as *mAs*. Mathematically this is simply expressed as follows: mA × s = mAs, where *s* represents exposure time in fractions of a second (as actual fractions or in decimal form) or in seconds. The quantity of electrons that flows from cathode to anode is directly proportionate to mAs (Box 2-6). The quantity of electrons that flows from cathode to anode is directly proportionate to the quantity of x-ray photons produced. An increase or decrease in mA, exposure time, or mAs directly affects the quantity of x-rays produced.

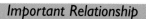

Important Relationship

The Quantity of Electrons, X-Rays, and mAs

The quantity of electrons flowing from the cathode to the anode and the quantity of x-rays produced are directly proportionate to mAs.

There is no effect of mAs on the quality of x-rays produced.

BOX 2-6 *mAs and X-Ray Quantity*

1. Higher mAs results in more electrons that move in the tube current from cathode to anode.
2. The more electrons in the tube current, the more x-rays that will be produced.
3. The number of x-rays that are produced is directly proportionate to the mAs.

Line Focus Principle

The **line focus principle** states that as the target angle decreases, so does the effective focal spot size.

Important Relationship

Line Focus Principle

The effective focal spot size decreases as the target angle decreases.

Focal spot size can be described in different ways. **Actual focal spot size** refers to the size of the area on the anode target that is being exposed to electrons from the tube current. **Effective focal spot size** refers to focal spot size as measured directly under the anode target. When an x-ray tube with a large target angle is used, a large actual focal spot size is produced and a large effective focal spot size is produced. When an x-ray tube with a small target angle is used, the same size actual focal spot size is produced but now a smaller effective focal spot size is produced. A small effective focal spot size will produce a radiograph with improved quality. The relationship among target angle, effective focal spot size, and actual focal spot size is illustrated in Figure 2-12. A smaller effective focal spot size can be achieved by using a smaller target angle. The actual focal spot size is the same as would be achieved with a larger target angle. Actual focal spot size depends on the size of the filament producing the electron stream that will interact with the anode target, not on the target angle. This is important because actual focal spot size, in part, determines the heat loading capacity of the x-ray tube. Smaller target angles produce better image quality without compromising the heat loading capacity of the tube.

Anode Heel Effect

A phenomenon known as the **anode heel effect** occurs because of the angle of the tube. The heel effect states that x-rays have a greater intensity on the cathode side of the tube, with the intensity diminishing toward the anode side (Figure 2-13).

Important Relationship

The Anode Heel Effect

X-rays are more intense on the cathode side of the tube. The intensity of the x-rays decreases toward the anode side.

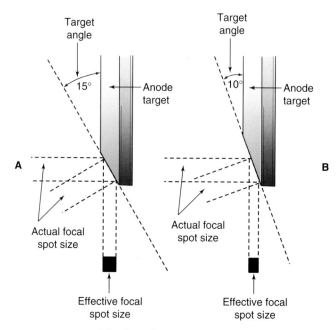

FIGURE 2-12 The line focus principle states that **(A)** a large target angle will produce a large effective focal spot size and that **(B)** a small target angle will produce a small effective focal spot size. Both actual focal spot sizes are the same, meaning that they can withstand the same heat loading from the same exposure factors.

X-rays that are emitted and directed toward the anode side of the beam are absorbed by the anode itself and are therefore reduced. The difference in the intensities between the two ends can be as much as 45%. The heel effect can be used to advantage in radiography because the cathode end of the tube can be placed over the thicker body part, resulting in more even density on the radiograph.

Beam Filtration

The x-ray beam produced at the anode must exit the tube housing to become the primary beam. This is the x-ray beam that will eventually record the body part onto the image receptor. The x-rays that exit the tube are polyenergetic. This means that they consist of low-, medium-, and high-energy photons. The low-energy photons do not contribute to image formation. They contribute only to patient dose.

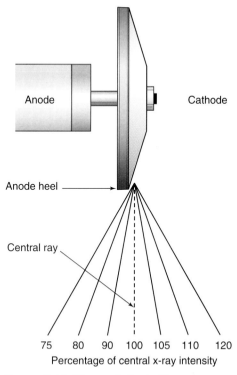

FIGURE 2-13 The anode heel effect.

Important Relationship

Low-Energy Photons, Patient Dose, and Image Formation

Low-energy photons contribute only to patient dose and not to image formation.

Reduction of the low-energy photons requires that filtration be added to the x-ray beam to attenuate, or absorb, these photons. **Added filtration** describes the filtration that is added to the port of the x-ray tube. Aluminum is the material primarily used for this purpose because it absorbs the low-energy photons while allowing the useful higher-energy photons to exit (Figure 2-14).

Various components within the x-ray tube assembly also contribute to the attenuation of low-energy x-rays. **Inherent filtration** refers to the filtration that is permanently in the path of the x-ray beam. Three components contribute to inherent filtration: (1) the glass envelope of the tube, (2) the oil that surrounds the tube, and (3) the mirror inside the collimator (Figure 2-14). **Total filtration** in the x-ray beam is the sum of the added filtration and the inherent filtration. The U.S. federal government sets minimum standards for total filtration to ensure that patients receive minimum

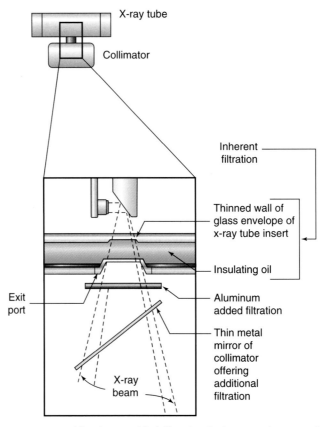

FIGURE 2-14 Aluminum-added filtration is shown at the port of the x-ray tube. The inherent filtration of the glass envelope, the oil, and the collimator mirror are shown.

doses of radiation. The current guidelines state that x-ray tubes operating above 70 kVp must have a minimum total filtration of 2.50 mm of aluminum or its equivalent.

HALF-VALUE LAYER

The **half-value layer (HVL)** is an indirect measure of the total filtration in the path of the x-ray beam. It is expressed in millimeters of aluminum (mm-Al). The HVL does not directly measure the total amount of aluminum in the x-ray beam. Instead, HVL is the amount of aluminum that is required to reduce the exposure to half its original value, assuming the kVp and mA remain fixed. The U.S. federal government specifies the minimum value of HVL for all diagnostic x-ray tubes. If the HVL is at the appropriate level, the total filtration in the x-ray tube is adequate to protect patients from unnecessary radiation.

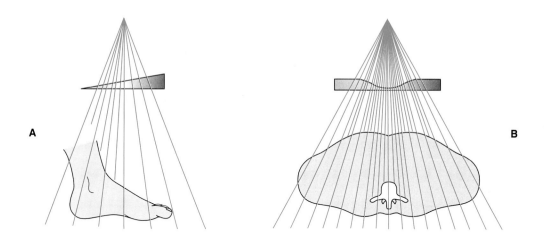

FIGURE 2-15 **A,** Wedge filter. **B,** Trough filter.

SPECIAL FILTERS

Special filters used in radiography can be added to the primary beam to alter its intensity. These types of filters assist in creating a radiographic image with more uniform density.

A **compensating filter** is a filter that is used to produce more uniform density on the radiographic image. The most common type of compensating filter is a simple **wedge filter** (Figure 2-15, *A*). The thicker part of the wedge filter is lined up with the less dense part of the body that is being imaged. The greater the angle of the wedge filter, the greater the change in x-ray intensity from one end to the other. A wedge filter is commonly used for an anteroposterior (AP) projection of the femur. A **trough filter** performs a function similar to the wedge filter; however, it is designed differently (Figure 2-15, *B*). The trough filter has a double wedge. A trough filter is commonly used for an AP projection of the thorax.

Heat Units

During x-ray production, most of the kinetic energy of the electrons is converted to heat. This heat can damage the x-ray tube and the anode target. The amount of heat produced with any given exposure is expressed by a unit called the **heat unit (HU).** The number of HUs produced depends on the type of x-ray generator being used and on the exposure factors selected for a particular procedure.

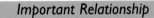

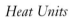

Important Relationship

Heat Units

The number of HUs produced depends on the type of x-ray generator used and the exposure factors selected.

Tube Rating Charts

Different models of x-ray tubes vary in their ability to withstand x-ray exposures in terms of the amount of heat produced. Manufacturers of x-ray tubes use instantaneous load tube rating charts, also called *single-exposure rating charts*, to describe the exposure limits of x-ray tubes. An **instantaneous load tube rating chart** is used to determine whether a particular exposure will be safe to make and to determine what limits on kVp, mA, and exposure time must be made to make a safe exposure. Violation of these limits as indicated by the tube rating chart will almost certainly result in permanent and irreparable damage to the x-ray tube. Figure 2-16 demonstrates a typical instantaneous load tube rating chart. For example, the maximum kVp that can be used with 700 mA and 0.3 second's exposure time is 90 kVp. The maximum mA that can be used with 105 kVp and 0.2 second's exposure time is 600 mA. The maximum exposure time that can be used with 85 kVp and 900 mA is 0.05 s. Whereas 130 kVp, 500 mA, and 0.1 s will produce a safe exposure, 130 kVp, 500 mA, and 0.2 s will not. Fortunately, manufacturers of x-ray machines build their equipment so that tube-damaging exposures cannot be made. Generally, if an inappropriate technique is set, the radiographer will see a message such as "Technique Overload," or the machine may simply not expose after the rotor button is activated.

Extending X-Ray Tube Life

X-ray tubes are expensive devices that can fail because of radiographer error or carelessness. Not only do failed tubes result in an expense for purchasing a new tube, but there is also down time for a radiographic room when a failed tube is being replaced, decreasing productivity of that room. A few simple but important guidelines of x-ray tube operation should be adhered to consistently by the radiographer to extend tube life.

- Warm up the tube according to the manufacturer's specifications. It is always important to refer to the manufacturer's guidelines when warming up the tube, but especially if it has not been energized for 2 hours or more.

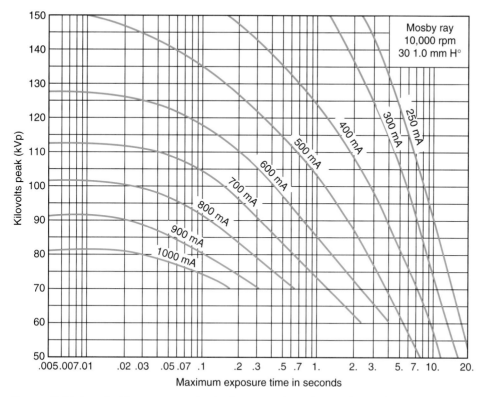

FIGURE 2-16 A typical instantaneous load tube rating chart that can be used to determine safe and unsafe exposures.

- Avoid excessive heat unit generation. Observe and heed the limits that the tube's rating chart places on the various combinations of kVp, mA, and exposure time. Figure 2-17 shows anode targets that have been damaged as a result of excessive heat loading.
- Do not hold down the rotor button without making an exposure. Holding down the rotor button unnecessarily causes excessive wear on both the filament and the rotor.
- Use lower tube currents with longer exposure times when possible. This will help minimize wear on the filament.
- Do not move the tube while it is energized. This movement can cause damage to the anode and anode stem as a result of torque, the force that acts to produce rotation.
- If the rotor makes noticeable noise, stop using the tube until it has been inspected by a qualified service person. Noises can be indicative of a potentially serious problem.

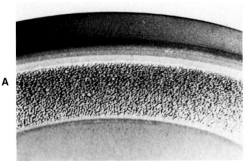
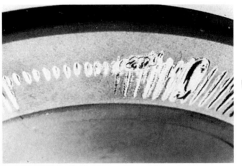

A   **B**

FIGURE 2-17 Two heat-damaged anode targets. Target **A** shows pitting of the anode track caused by consistent overloading of exposure factors. Target **B** shows melting of the focal track caused by failure of the rotor to rotate the anode. This failure usually results from heat damage of the rotor bearings from overloading the exposure factors. *Courtesy Varian Interay.*

Radiographers create diagnostic images by producing an x-ray beam that provides visualization of anatomic structures. The x-rays produced by the radiographer affect not only the quality of the image but also the life of the x-ray tube. Understanding the prime exposure factors and their effect on the x-ray beam and knowing what happens inside the x-ray tube are important considerations in radiography.

REVIEW QUESTIONS

1. Which x-ray tube component serves as a source of electrons for x-ray production?
   A. Focusing cup
   B. Filament
   C. Stator
   D. Target

2. Electrons interact with the _____ to produce x-rays and heat.
   A. focusing cup
   B. filament
   C. stator
   D. target

3. The cloud of electrons that forms before x-ray production is referred to as
   A. thermionic emission.
   B. space charge.
   C. space charge effect.
   D. tube current.

4. The burning off of electrons at the cathode is referred to as
   A. thermionic emission.
   B. space charge.
   C. space charge effect.
   D. tube current.

5. Which primary exposure factor influences both the quantity and the quality of x-ray photons?
   A. mA
   B. mAs
   C. kVp
   D. Exposure time

6. The unit used to express tube current is
   A. mA
   B. mAs
   C. kVp
   D. s

7. What percentage of the kinetic energy is converted to heat when moving electrons strike the anode target?
  A. 1%
  B. 25%
  C. 59%
  D. 99%

8. The intensity of the x-ray beam is greater on the
  A. cathode side of the tube.
  B. anode side of the tube.
  C. short axis of the beam.
  D. long axis of the beam.

9. According to the line focus principle, as the target angle decreases, the
  A. actual focal spot size decreases.
  B. actual focal spot size increases.
  C. effective focal spot size decreases.
  D. effective focal spot size increases.

10. _____ will extend x-ray tube life.
  A. Selecting higher tube currents
  B. Using the small focal spot when possible
  C. Producing exposures with a wide range of kVp values
  D. Warming up the tube after 2 hours of nonuse

CHAPTER 3

Radiographic Image Formation

DIFFERENTIAL ABSORPTION

Beam Attenuation
    Absorption
    Scattering
    Transmission
    Exit Radiation

REVIEW QUESTIONS

OBJECTIVES

1 Define all of the key terms in this chapter.

2 State all of the important relationships in this chapter.

3 Describe the process of radiographic image formation.

4 Explain the process of beam attenuation.

5 Describe the x-ray interactions termed *photoelectric effect* and *Compton effect*.

6 Define the term *ionization*.

7 State the composition of exit radiation.

8 State the effect of scatter radiation on the radiographic image.

9 Explain the process of creating the various shades of radiographic densities

KEY TERMS

image receptor
differential absorption
attenuation
absorption
photoelectron
ionization
photoelectric effect
scattering

Compton effect
Compton electron/secondary electron
transmission
exit radiation
fog
latent/invisible image
manifest/visible image

To produce a radiographic image, x-ray photons must pass through tissue and interact with an **image receptor** (a device that receives the radiation leaving the patient), such as a film-screen system. Both the quantity and quality of the primary x-ray beam will affect its interaction within the various tissues that make up the anatomic part. In addition, the composition of the anatomic tissues will affect the x-ray beam interaction. The absorption characteristics of the anatomic part are determined by its composition, such as thickness, atomic number, and compactness of the cellular structures. Last, the radiation that exits the patient will do so in varying energies, causing different shades of gray on the image receptor after processing.

Differential Absorption

The process of image formation where the x-ray beam interacts with the anatomic tissue and a portion of the beam strikes the image receptor is a result of **differential absorption.** Differential absorption is a process whereby some of the x-ray beam will be absorbed in the tissue and some will pass through (transmit) the anatomic part. The term *differential* is used because varying anatomic parts do not *absorb* the primary beam the same. Anatomic parts composed of bone will absorb more x-ray photons than parts filled with air. Differential absorption of the primary x-ray beam will create an image that structurally represents the anatomic area of interest (Figure 3-1).

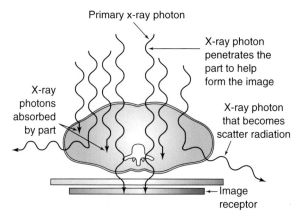

Primary x-ray photon

X-ray photon penetrates the part to help form the image

X-ray photons absorbed by part

X-ray photon that becomes scatter radiation

Image receptor

FIGURE 3-1 As the primary x-ray beam interacts with the anatomic part, photons will be absorbed, scattered, and transmitted. The differences in the absorption characteristics of the anatomic part create an image that structurally represents the anatomic part.

Differential Absorption and Image Formation

A radiographic image is created by passing an x-ray beam through the patient and interacting with an image receptor, such as a film-screen system. The variations in absorption and transmission of the exiting x-ray beam will structurally represent the anatomic area of interest.

Creating a radiographic image by differential absorption requires that several processes occur.

BEAM ATTENUATION

As the primary x-ray beam passes through anatomic tissue, it will lose some of its energy. This reduction in the energy of the primary x-ray beam is known as **attenuation.** Beam attenuation occurs as a result of the photon interactions with the atomic structures that compose the tissues. Three distinct processes occur during beam attenuation: absorption, scattering, and photon transmission.

Absorption

As the energy of the primary x-ray beam is deposited within the atoms composing the tissue, some x-ray photons will be completely absorbed. Complete **absorption** of the incoming x-ray photon occurs when it has enough energy to remove (eject) an inner-shell electron. The ejected electron is called a **photoelectron.** The ability to remove (eject) electrons, known as **ionization,** is one of the characteristics of x-rays. In the diagnostic range, this x-ray interaction with matter is known as the **photoelectric effect.**

With the photoelectric effect, the ionized atom has a vacancy, or electron hole, in its inner shell. An electron from an upper-level shell will drop down to fill the vacancy. As a result of the difference in binding energies between the two electron shells, a secondary x-ray photon will be emitted (Figure 3-2). This secondary x-ray photon is a form of scatter radiation and may exit the patient or interact with other tissue electrons.

X-Ray Photon Absorption

During attenuation of the x-ray beam, the photoelectric effect is responsible for total absorption of the incoming x-ray photon.

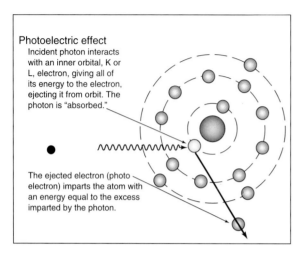

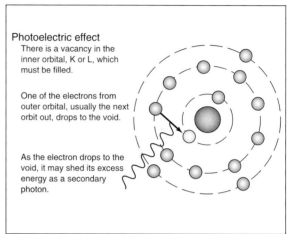

FIGURE 3-2 The photoelectric effect is responsible for total absorption of the incoming x-ray photon.

Whether the incoming photon is totally absorbed depends on its energy and the atomic number of the anatomic tissue. After absorption of some of the x-ray photons, the overall energy of the primary beam will be decreased as it passes through the anatomic part.

Scattering

Some incoming photons will not be absorbed, but instead they will lose energy during interactions with the atoms composing the tissue. This process is called **scattering** and results from the diagnostic x-ray interaction with matter known as the **Compton effect.** The loss of energy of the incoming photon occurs when it ejects an outer-shell electron from the atom. The ejected electron is called a **Compton electron** or **secondary electron.** The remaining lower-energy x-ray photon will change direction and may leave the anatomic part to interact with the image receptor (Figure 3-3).

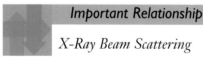

Important Relationship

X-Ray Beam Scattering

During attenuation of the x-ray beam, the incoming x-ray photon may lose energy and change direction as a result of the Compton effect.

If a scattered photon strikes the image receptor, it will not contribute any useful information regarding the anatomic area of interest. If scattered photons are

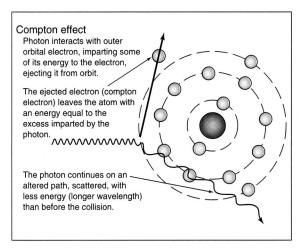

Compton effect
Photon interacts with outer orbital electron, imparting some of its energy to the electron, ejecting it from orbit.

The ejected electron (compton electron) leaves the atom with an energy equal to the excess imparted by the photon.

The photon continues on an altered path, scattered, with less energy (longer wavelength) than before the collision.

FIGURE 3-3 During the Compton effect, the incoming photon loses energy and changes its direction.

absorbed within the anatomic tissue, they will contribute to the radiation exposure to the patient. In addition, if the scattered photon leaves the patient and does not strike the image receptor, it could contribute to the radiation exposure of anyone within close proximity to the patient.

The probability of a Compton interaction occurring is not dependent on the energy of the incoming photon or the composition of the anatomic tissue. Compton interactions can occur within all diagnostic x-ray energies and are therefore an important interaction in radiography. Scattered and secondary radiations provide no useful information and must be controlled during radiographic imaging.

The preceding discussion focused on photon interactions that occur in radiography when using x-ray energies within the moderate range. Lower- and higher-energy x-rays result in other interactions (classic or coherent scattering, pair production, and photodisintegration) when the x-ray energies are beyond the moderate range used in radiography.

Transmission

If the incoming x-ray photon passes through the anatomic part without any interaction with the atomic structures, it is called **transmission** (Figure 3-4). The combination of absorption and transmission of the x-ray beam will provide an image that structurally represents the anatomic part. Because scatter radiation is also a process that occurs during interaction of the x-ray beam and anatomic part, the quality of the image created will be compromised if the scattered photon strikes the image receptor.

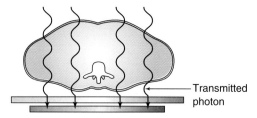

FIGURE 3-4 Some incoming x-ray photons will pass through the anatomic part without any interactions.

Practical Tip

X-Ray Interaction with Matter

When the primary x-ray beam interacts with anatomic tissues, three processes occur during attenuation of the x-ray beam: absorption, scattering, and transmission.

Exit Radiation

When the attenuated x-ray beam leaves the patient, the remaining x-ray beam, referred to as **exit radiation,** is composed of both transmitted and scattered radiation (Figure 3-5). The varying amounts of transmitted and absorbed radiation (differential absorption) will create an image that structurally represents the anatomic area of interest. Scatter exit radiation that reaches the image receptor will not provide any diagnostic information about the anatomic area. Scatter radiation creates unwanted density on the image called **fog.** Methods used to decrease the amount of scatter radiation reaching the image receptor are discussed in later chapters.

The areas within the anatomic tissue that absorb incoming x-ray photons will create the white or clear areas (low density) on the radiographic image. The incoming x-ray photons that are transmitted will create the black areas (high density) on the radiographic image. Anatomic tissues that vary in absorption and transmission will create a range of dark and light areas (shades of gray) (Figure 3-6).

Important Relationship

Image Densities

The range of image densities are created by the variation in x-ray absorption and transmission as the x-ray beam passes through anatomic tissues.

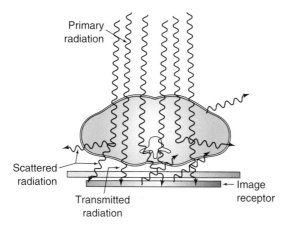

Primary radiation

Scattered radiation

Transmitted radiation

Image receptor

FIGURE 3-5 Radiation that exits the anatomic part comprises transmitted and scattered radiation.

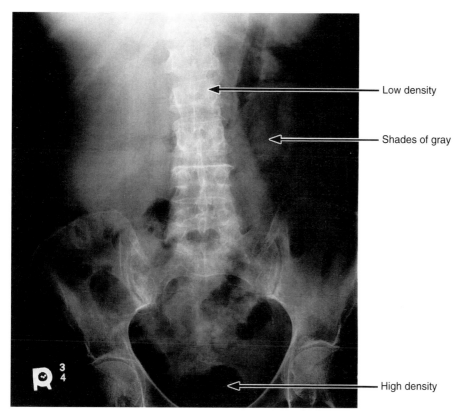

Low density

Shades of gray

High density

FIGURE 3-6 A radiographic image represents the various absorption characteristics of the anatomic part. An area of high density is where the x-ray beam was transmitted, and an area of low density is where the x-ray beam was absorbed. Anatomic tissues that vary in absorption and transmission create the shades of gray on the image.

The exit radiation that interacts with an image receptor, such as a film-screen system, will create the **latent** or **invisible image.** This latent image will not be visible until the exposed film is developed and processed to produce the **manifest** or **visible image.**

Several important steps in creating a radiographic image have been discussed in this and the previous chapters. Further discussion of radiographic image quality, image receptors, control of scatter radiation, exposure technique selection, and problem solving are included in subsequent chapters.

Review Questions

1. The process whereby a radiographic image is created by passing an x-ray beam through anatomic tissue is known as
   A. attenuation.
   B. the photoelectric effect.
   C. the Compton effect.
   D. differential absorption.

2. Which of the following processes occurs during beam attenuation: 1.) absorption, 2.) photon transmission, or 3.) scattering?
   A. 1 and 2 only
   B. 1 and 3 only
   C. 2 and 3 only
   D. 1, 2, and 3

3. The ability of an x-ray photon to remove an atom's electron is a characteristic known as
   A. attenuation.
   B. scattering.
   C. ionization.
   D. absorption.

4. The x-ray interaction responsible for absorption is
   A. differential.
   B. photoelectric.
   C. attenuation.
   D. Compton.

5. The x-ray interaction responsible for scattering is
   A. differential.
   B. photoelectric.
   C. attenuation.
   D. Compton.

6. Exit radiation is composed of which of the following: 1.) transmitted radiation, 2.) absorbed radiation, or 3.) scattered radiation?
   A. 1 and 2 only
   B. 1 and 3 only
   C. 2 and 3 only
   D. 1, 2, and 3

7. What interaction creates unwanted density known as fog?
   A. Compton
   B. Transmitted
   C. Photoelectric
   D. Absorption

8. The low-density areas on a radiographic image are created by
   A. transmitted radiation.
   B. scattered radiation.
   C. absorbed radiation.
   D. primary radiation.

9. An anatomic part that transmits the incoming x-ray photon will create an area of _____ on the radiographic image.
   A. fog
   B. low density
   C. high density
   D. gray

10. Development and processing of an exposed film will result in a(n)
    A. manifest image.
    B. latent image.
    C. invisible image.
    D. inert image.

CHAPTER 4

Radiographic Image Quality

PHOTOGRAPHIC PROPERTIES (VISIBILITY)

Radiographic Density
   Controlling Factors
   Influencing Factors
Radiographic Contrast
   Controlling Factor
   Influencing Factors

GEOMETRIC PROPERTIES (SHARPNESS)

Recorded Detail
   Geometric Unsharpness
   Image Receptor Unsharpness
   Measuring Recorded Detail
   Motion Unsharpness
Distortion
   Size Distortion (Magnification)
   Shape Distortion

FILM CRITIQUE

REVIEW QUESTIONS

OBJECTIVES

1 Define all of the key terms in this chapter.

2 State all of the important relationships in this chapter.

3 Define the necessary components of radiographic image quality.

4 Differentiate between the photographic and geometric properties of a radiograph.

5 Differentiate among an optimal, diagnostic, and unacceptable radiograph.

6 Define *radiographic density* and discuss the controlling and influencing factors.

7 State how mAs and kVp can be used to adjust a density error.

8 Calculate changes in mAs and kVp to adjust radiographic density.

9 Define *radiographic contrast* and discuss the controlling and influencing factors.

10 Calculate changes in kVp to adjust radiographic contrast.

11 Explain the methods used to obtain a desired level of radiographic contrast.

12 Discuss the importance of both density and contrast in the visibility of recorded detail.

13 Define *recorded detail* and discuss the factors affecting geometric unsharpness, receptor unsharpness, and motion unsharpness.

14 Using the geometric unsharpness formula, calculate the changes in the amount of unsharpness when varying SID, OID, and focal spot size.

15 Define *distortion* and discuss the factors that affect both the size and the shape of the recorded image.

16 Calculate the magnification factor and determine the changes in the image and/or object size.

17 Discuss the importance of both the visibility and sharpness of recorded detail in producing a quality radiographic image.

KEY TERMS

visibility of recorded detail (photographic properties)
sharpness of recorded detail (geometric properties)
radiographic density
15% rule
inverse square law
density maintenance formula
anode heel effect
reciprocity law
radiographic contrast
high contrast
short-scale contrast
low contrast
long-scale contrast

film (image receptor) contrast
subject contrast
contrast medium
geometric properties
recorded detail
geometric unsharpness
resolution
blur
distortion
size distortion/magnification
magnification factor (MF)
source-to-object distance (SOD)
elongation
foreshortening

A primary responsibility of the radiographer is to evaluate radiographic images to determine whether sufficient information exists for a diagnosis. Evaluating radiographic quality requires the radiographer to assess the image for both its **visibility of recorded detail (photographic properties)** and its **sharpness of recorded detail (geometric properties).** Radiographic quality is the combination of both the visibility and the sharpness of recorded detail. The radiographer must be knowledgeable about the factors that affect the photographic and geometric properties of a radiographic image to produce radiographs of optimal quality (Figure 4-1).

Photographic Properties (Visibility)

Photographic properties (visibility factors) of recorded detail are the extent to which the structural components of the anatomic area of interest can be seen on the recorded image. The radiographer views the entire image to determine whether the recorded detail is visualized sufficiently. When the radiographer determines that the visibility of recorded detail is maximized, the image is of optimal photographic quality. If the radiographer determines that the visibility of recorded detail is adequate or acceptable, the image is of diagnostic photographic quality. In the event that the radiographer determines the recorded detail is not adequately visualized, the image is unacceptable and the study must be repeated. At this point, the radiographer must problem solve to determine the factors that need to be adjusted to improve the visualization of the recorded detail. Visibility of the recorded detail is achieved by the proper balance of radiographic density and radiographic contrast.

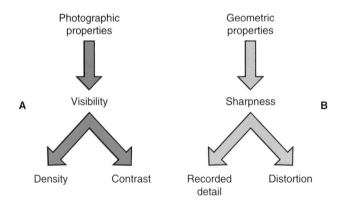

FIGURE 4-1 Factors affecting radiographic image quality. **A,** Photographic properties. **B,** Geometric properties.

RADIOGRAPHIC DENSITY

Radiographic density is the amount of overall blackness produced on the image after processing. A radiograph must have sufficient density to visualize the anatomic structures of interest (Figure 4-2). A radiograph that is too light has insufficient density to visualize the structures of the anatomic part (Figure 4-3). Conversely, a radiograph that is too dark has excessive density, and the anatomic part will not be well visualized (Figure 4-4). The radiographer must evaluate the overall density on the radiograph to determine whether it is sufficient to visualize the anatomic area of interest. He or she will then decide whether the radiograph is optimal, diagnostic, or unacceptable. The ability to determine when a radiograph is unacceptable as a result of either insufficient or excessive density requires knowledge of the radiographic factors and clinical experience.

If a radiograph is deemed unacceptable, the radiographer must problem solve to determine what factors contributed to the density error. Knowledge about the factors that affect the density on a radiograph is critical to developing strong problem-solving skills. Factors that directly affect density are identified as controlling factors, whereas influencing factors indirectly affect density (Box 4-1).

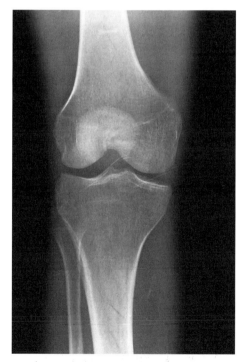

FIGURE 4-2 Radiograph with optimal density. *From* Mosby's instructional radiographic series: radiographic imaging, *St Louis, 1998, Mosby.*

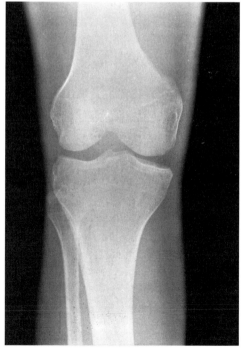

FIGURE 4-3 Radiograph with insufficient density. *From* Mosby's instructional radiographic series: radiographic imaging, *St Louis, 1998, Mosby.*

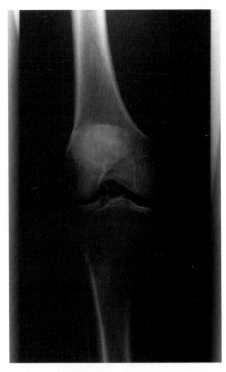

FIGURE 4-4 Radiograph with excessive density.

BOX 4-1 *Factors Affecting Density*

Controlling Factors
Milliamperage
Exposure time

Influencing Factors
Kilovoltage
Distance
Grids
Film-screen speed
Collimation
Anatomic part
Anode heel effect
Reciprocity law
Generator output
Tube filtration
Film processing

Controlling Factors

The quantity of radiation reaching the image receptor has a primary effect on the amount of radiographic density produced (Box 4-2).

Box 4-2 *Controlling Factors for Radiographic Density*

Milliamperage and exposure time control the quantity of radiation reaching the image receptor.

As you recall from Chapter 2, the product of milliamperage (mA) and exposure time (mAs) has a direct proportional relationship with the quantity of x-rays produced. When the quantity of x-rays is increased, the radiographic density also increases. Conversely, when the quantity of x-rays is decreased, the radiographic density decreases. Therefore radiographic density can be increased or decreased by adjusting the quantity of radiation (mAs).

Important Relationship

mAs, Quantity of Radiation, and Radiographic Density

As the mAs is increased, the quantity of radiation is increased and radiographic density is increased. As the mAs is decreased, the quantity of radiation is decreased and radiographic density is decreased.

Because mAs is the product of milliamperage and exposure time, increasing milliamperage or time will have the same effect on density.

Mathematical Application

Adjusting Milliamperage, Exposure Time, or Both to Control Density

100 mA @ 0.10 s = 10 mAs. To increase the mAs to 20, you could use:

$$200 \text{ mA @ } 0.10 \text{ s} = 20 \text{ mAs}$$
$$100 \text{ mA @ } 0.20 \text{ s} = 20 \text{ mAs}$$
$$400 \text{ mA @ } 0.05 \text{ s} = 20 \text{ mAs}$$

As demonstrated in the mathematical application, mAs can be doubled by doubling the milliamperage or doubling the exposure time. A change in either milliamperage or exposure time will proportionally change the mAs. To maintain the same mAs, the radiographer must increase the milliamperage and proportionally decrease the exposure time.

Important Relationship

Milliamperage and Exposure Time

Milliamperage and exposure time have an inverse relationship when maintaining the same mAs.

A change in mAs results in a direct change in density. For example, when the mAs is increased, density is increased; when the mAs is decreased, density is decreased (Figure 4-5).

When a radiograph is too light (insufficient density), a greater increase in mAs may be needed to correct the density, or the mAs may need to be decreased by more to correct a radiograph that has excessive density. This relationship between the quantity of radiation and density is discussed in more detail in Chapter 8.

The challenge for radiographers is to assess the level of density produced on a radiograph and to determine whether the amount of density needs adjustment. When a radiograph is deemed unacceptable and the study must be repeated, the radiographer must then decide how much of a change in mAs is needed to correct for the density error.

In general, for repeats that are necessary because of density errors, the mAs is adjusted by a factor of 2; therefore a minimum change made for a repeat is to double or halve the mAs. As mentioned previously, it may take more than doubling the mAs to correct for a density error. If the radiograph needs more adjustment than a factor of 2, the radiographer should multiply or divide the mAs by 4 (Figure 4-6).

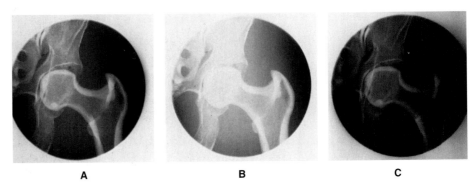

A   B   C

FIGURE 4-5 Changes in mAs have a direct effect on density. **A** is the original image. **B** shows the decrease in density when the mAs is decreased by half. **C** shows the increase in density when the mAs is doubled.

Repeating Radiographs Because of Density Errors

The minimum change needed to correct for a density error is determined by multiplying or dividing the mAs by 2. When a greater change in mAs is needed, the radiographer should multiply or divide by 4, 8, and so on.

Radiographs that have sufficient but not optimal density usually are not repeated. If a radiograph must be repeated because of another error, such as positioning, the radiographer may also use the opportunity to make an adjustment in density to produce a radiograph of optimal quality. Making a visible change in radiographic density requires that the minimum amount of change in mAs be approximately 30% (depending on equipment, somewhere between 25% and 35%). Remember, radiographic studies generally are not repeated for only a visible change in density. A radiographic study repeated because of insufficient or excessive density requires a change in mAs by a factor of at least 2.

Influencing Factors

Although mAs is the controlling factor for radiographic density, other factors also affect density (see Box 4-1).

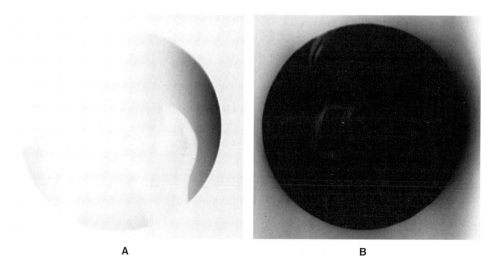

A   B

FIGURE 4-6 **A** needs a greater increase in mAs, four times the original mAs. **B** needs a greater decrease in mAs, one-fourth the original mAs.

Increasing the kVp by 15% increases the radiographic density, unless the mAs is decreased. Also, decreasing the kVp by 15% decreases the radiographic density, unless the mAs is increased. As mentioned earlier, the effect of changes in kVp is not uniform throughout the range of kVp. When low or high kilovoltages are used, the amount of change in kVp required to maintain the density may be greater or less than 15%.

X   Mathematical Application

Using the 15% Rule

To increase density: Multiply the kVp by 1.15 (original kVp + 15%).

$$80 \text{ kVp} \times 1.15 = 92 \text{ kVp}$$

To decrease density: Multiply the kVp by 0.85 (original kVp − 15%).

$$80 \text{ kVp} \times 0.85 = 68 \text{ kVp}$$

To maintain density:

When increasing kVp by 15% (kVp × 1.15), divide the original mAs by 2.

$$80 \text{ kVp} \times 1.15 = 92 \text{ kVp and mAs/2}$$

When decreasing the kVp by 15% (kVp × 0.85), multiply the mAs by 2.

$$80 \text{ kVp} \times 0.85 = 68 \text{ kVp and mAs} \times 2$$

Distance

The distance between the source of the radiation and the image receptor (source-to-image receptor distance [SID]) affects the amount of density produced on a radiograph. Because of the divergence of the x-ray beam, the intensity of the radiation will vary at different distances. This relationship between distance and x-ray beam intensity is best described by the **inverse square law,** which states that the intensity of the x-ray beam is inversely proportionate to the square of the distance from the source. Because beam intensity varies as a function of the square of the distance, SID affects the quantity of radiation reaching the image receptor. As SID increases, density decreases; as SID decreases, density increases.

Important Relationship

SID and Radiographic Density

As SID increases, the radiographic density decreases as a result of the square of the distance. As SID decreases, the radiographic density increases as a result of the square of the distance.

The minimum change needed to correct for a density error is determined by multiplying or dividing the mAs by 2. When a greater change in mAs is needed, the radiographer should multiply or divide by 4, 8, and so on.

Radiographs that have sufficient but not optimal density usually are not repeated. If a radiograph must be repeated because of another error, such as positioning, the radiographer may also use the opportunity to make an adjustment in density to produce a radiograph of optimal quality. Making a visible change in radiographic density requires that the minimum amount of change in mAs be approximately 30% (depending on equipment, somewhere between 25% and 35%). Remember, radiographic studies generally are not repeated for only a visible change in density. A radiographic study repeated because of insufficient or excessive density requires a change in mAs by a factor of at least 2.

Influencing Factors

Although mAs is the controlling factor for radiographic density, other factors also affect density (see Box 4-1).

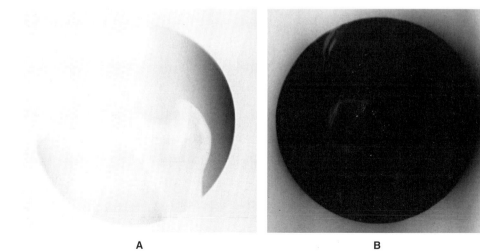

A   **B**

FIGURE 4-6 **A** needs a greater increase in mAs, four times the original mAs. **B** needs a greater decrease in mAs, one-fourth the original mAs.

Kilovoltage

Kilovoltage peak (kVp) affects radiographic density because it alters the amount and penetrating ability of the x-ray beam. Increasing the penetration of the x-ray beam results in more radiation reaching the image receptor. As a result, more density is produced on the radiographic image (Figure 4-7).

Important Relationship

Kilovoltage and Radiographic Density

Increasing the kilovoltage peak increases the quantity of radiation reaching the image receptor and therefore increases radiographic density. Decreasing the kilovoltage peak decreases the quantity of radiation reaching the image receptor and therefore decreases radiographic density.

However, the effect of kilovoltage peak (kVp) on density is not proportional. In addition, the effect of kVp on density will not be equal throughout the range of kilovoltage (low, middle, and high). A greater change in kVp is needed when operating at a high kVp (greater than 90) compared with operating at a low kVp (less than 70) (Figure 4-8).

Kilovoltage affects not only the amount of density but also other aspects of the image; therefore kilovoltage is not the primary factor to manipulate for changes in radiographic density. However, it is sometimes necessary to manipulate the kilovoltage to maintain or adjust the density.

Maintaining or adjusting radiographic density can be accomplished with kilovoltage by using the **15% rule.** The 15% rule states that changing the kilovoltage peak

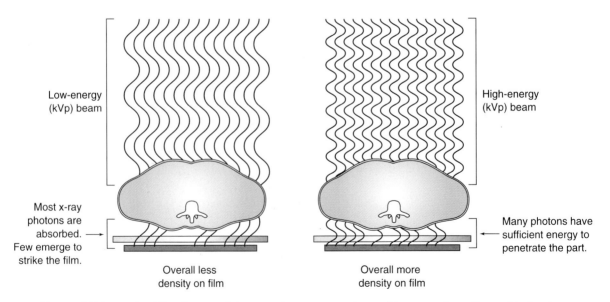

Low-energy (kVp) beam

High-energy (kVp) beam

Most x-ray photons are absorbed. Few emerge to strike the film.

Many photons have sufficient energy to penetrate the part.

Overall less density on film

Overall more density on film

FIGURE 4-7 Increasing kilovoltage peak increases beam penetration and increases the radiographic density.

by 15% will have the same effect on radiographic density as doubling the mAs, or reducing the mAs by 50%; for example, increasing the kilovoltage peak from 82 to 92 (15%) will have the same effect on density as increasing the mAs from 10 to 20. Increasing the kilovoltage by 15% will increase the density by 2, and decreasing the kilovoltage by 15% will decrease the density by half.

 Practical Tip

Kilovoltage and the 15% Rule

A 15% increase in kilovoltage peak will have the same effect on radiographic density as doubling the mAs. A 15% decrease in kVp will have the same effect on radiographic density as decreasing the mAs by half.

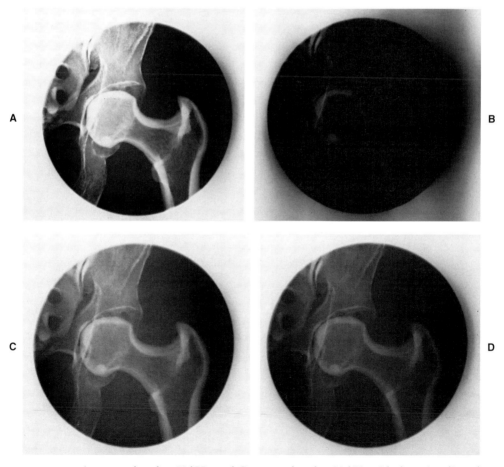

FIGURE 4-8 **A** was produced at 50 kVp, and **C** was produced at 90 kVp with the mAs adjusted to maintain radiographic density. A 10-kVp increase at 50 kVp **(B)** will produce a greater change in density than a 10-kVp increase at 90 kVp **(D).**

Increasing the kVp by 15% increases the radiographic density, unless the mAs is decreased. Also, decreasing the kVp by 15% decreases the radiographic density, unless the mAs is increased. As mentioned earlier, the effect of changes in kVp is not uniform throughout the range of kVp. When low or high kilovoltages are used, the amount of change in kVp required to maintain the density may be greater or less than 15%.

 X *Mathematical Application*

Using the 15% Rule

To increase density: Multiply the kVp by 1.15 (original kVp + 15%).

80 kVp × 1.15 = 92 kVp

To decrease density: Multiply the kVp by 0.85 (original kVp − 15%).

80 kVp × 0.85 = 68 kVp

To maintain density:

When increasing kVp by 15% (kVp × 1.15), divide the original mAs by 2.

80 kVp × 1.15 = 92 kVp and mAs/2

When decreasing the kVp by 15% (kVp × 0.85), multiply the mAs by 2.

80 kVp × 0.85 = 68 kVp and mAs × 2

Distance

The distance between the source of the radiation and the image receptor (source-to-image receptor distance [SID]) affects the amount of density produced on a radiograph. Because of the divergence of the x-ray beam, the intensity of the radiation will vary at different distances. This relationship between distance and x-ray beam intensity is best described by the **inverse square law,** which states that the intensity of the x-ray beam is inversely proportionate to the square of the distance from the source. Because beam intensity varies as a function of the square of the distance, SID affects the quantity of radiation reaching the image receptor. As SID increases, density decreases; as SID decreases, density increases.

 Important Relationship

SID and Radiographic Density

As SID increases, the radiographic density decreases as a result of the square of the distance. As SID decreases, the radiographic density increases as a result of the square of the distance.

Maintaining consistent densities when the SID is altered requires that the mAs be adjusted to compensate. The **density maintenance formula** (also known as *mAs/distance compensation formula*) provides a mathematical calculation for adjusting the mAs to change the SID.

X Mathematical Application

Density Maintenance Formula

$$\frac{mAs_1}{mAs_2} = \frac{(SID)^2_1}{(SID)^2_2}$$

For example, optimal density is achieved at an SID of 40 inches using 25 mAs. The SID must be increased to 56 inches. What adjustment in mAs is needed to maintain radiographic density?

$$\frac{25}{mAs_2} = \frac{(40)^2}{(56)^2}; \ 1600 \times = 78,400; \ \frac{78,400}{1600}; \ mAs_2 = 49$$

Because increasing the SID decreases the density, the mAs must be increased accordingly to maintain density. When the SID is decreased, the density increases; therefore the mAs must be decreased accordingly to maintain density.

Important Relationship

SID and mAs

Increasing the SID requires that mAs be increased to maintain density, and decreasing the SID requires a decrease in mAs to maintain density.

Standard distances are used in radiography to provide more consistency in radiographic quality. Most diagnostic radiography is performed at an SID of 40, 48, or 72 inches. Certain circumstances, such as trauma or mobile radiography, do not allow for standard distances to be used. In these circumstances the radiographer must determine the change needed in the mAs to obtain a radiograph with adequate density.

Practical Tip

Altering SID between 40 and 72 Inches

When a 72-inch SID cannot be used, adjusting the SID to 56 inches requires half the mAs. When a 40-inch SID cannot be used, adjusting the SID to 56 inches requires twice the mAs. This quick method of calculating mAs changes should produce sufficient density.

Grids

A radiographic grid is a device that is placed between the patient and the image receptor to absorb scatter radiation exiting the patient. Limiting the amount of scatter radiation that reaches the image receptor improves the quality of the radiograph. Grids also absorb some of the transmitted radiation exiting the patient and therefore reduce the amount of density produced on a radiograph.

Important Relationship

Grids and Radiographic Density

Adding, removing, or changing a grid requires an adjustment in mAs to maintain radiographic density.

When grids are used, the mAs must be adjusted to maintain sufficient density. In addition, the more efficient a grid is in absorbing scatter, the greater the increase in mAs required to maintain the density. The grid conversion formula is a mathematical formula for adjusting the mAs for changes in the type of grid (Table 4-1).

When a grid is added, the radiographer must use the correct grid conversion factor to multiply by the mAs to compensate for the decreased density. When a grid is removed, the correct conversion grid factor must be divided into the mAs to compensate for the increased density. When the grid ratio is changed, the following formula should be used to adjust the density:

$$\frac{mAs_1}{mAs_2} = \frac{Grid\ conversion\ factor_2}{Grid\ conversion\ factor_1}$$

The new mAs will produce a density comparable to that of the original exposure technique.

TABLE 4-1   GRID CONVERSION CHART

Grid Ratios	Grid Conversion Factor
5:1	2×
6:1	3×
8:1	4×
12:1	5×
16:1	6×

Grids primarily are used to increase radiographic contrast and are discussed later in this chapter. The construction, conversion formula, and use of grids are discussed in more detail in Chapter 5.

Film-Screen Speed

The combination of the film and intensifying screen will affect the image receptor's sensitivity to radiation exposure. The more sensitive the film-screen system is to radiation, the faster the speed. The speed of the film-screen system affects the amount of radiation required to produce a given amount of radiographic density. The greater the speed, the greater the density.

Important Relationship

Film-Screen System Speed and Radiographic Density

The greater the speed of the film-screen system, the greater the amount of density produced on the radiograph; the lower the speed of the film-screen system, the less density produced on the radiograph.

Because the film-screen system speed affects radiographic density, the mAs needs to be adjusted if the film-screen speed is changed. Increasing the film-screen system speed requires a decrease to be made to the mAs to maintain radiographic density. A decrease in the film-screen system speed requires an increase to be made to the mAs to maintain density.

Important Relationship

Film-Screen System Speed and mAs

Increasing the film-screen speed requires a decrease to be made to the mAs to maintain density, and decreasing the film-screen speed requires an increase to be made to the mAs to maintain density.

Film-screen systems are classified by their relative speed (RS) factor. Film-screen relative speeds range from 50 RS to as high as 800 RS. Extremity film-screen combinations usually have an RS of 100, and routine high-speed film-screen combinations have an RS of 400. The RS classification for film-screen systems provides a method whereby exposure techniques can be adjusted for changes in film-screen speed.

The relative film-screen speed conversion formula is a mathematical formula for adjusting the mAs for changes in the film-screen system speed.

$$\frac{mAs_1}{mAs_2} = \frac{RS_2}{RS_1}$$

The correct relative film-screen speed factors must be used to calculate the new mAs required to compensate for changes in density. The new mAs will produce a density comparable to that of the original exposure technique. Construction of films and intensifying screens and the screen conversion formula are discussed further in Chapter 6.

Collimation

Any changes in the size of the x-ray field will alter the amount of tissue irradiated. Increasing the field size (less collimation) increases the amount of tissue irradiated and increases the amount of scatter radiation reaching the image receptor, which in turn increases the amount of density on the radiograph. Conversely, decreasing the field size (more collimation) reduces the amount of tissue irradiated and the amount of scatter radiation reaching the image receptor. This decrease will reduce the amount of density on the radiograph.

The effect of collimation on the radiographic density is more visible when imaging large anatomic areas, performing examinations without a grid, and using a high kilovoltage.

Anatomic Part

The thickness of the anatomic part being imaged affects the amount of x-ray beam attenuation that occurs. A thick part absorbs more radiation, whereas a thin part transmits more radiation.

Important Relationship

Part Thickness and Radiographic Density

A thick anatomic part decreases the radiographic density. A thin anatomic part increases radiographic density.

Maintaining density when imaging a thicker part requires the mAs to be increased accordingly. In addition, when a thinner anatomic part is being radiographed, the mAs must be decreased accordingly.

In general, for every change in part thickness of 4 cm, the radiographer should adjust the mAs by a factor of 2.

X *Mathematical Application*

Adjusting mAs for Changes in Part Thickness

An optimal radiograph was obtained using 40 mAs on an anatomic part that measured 18 cm. The same anatomic part is radiographed in another patient, and it measures 22 cm. What new mAs is needed to maintain density? Because the part thickness was increased by 4 cm, the original mAs is multiplied by 2, yielding 80 mAs.

In addition to part thickness, many disease processes change the absorption characteristics of the anatomic area. Additive disease processes (increased tissue) increase the absorption of the x-ray beam and require an increase in the exposure technique. Destructive disease processes (decreased tissue) decrease the absorption of the x-ray beam and require a decrease in the exposure technique.

Determining the extent of the additive or destructive disease is difficult. Unless the radiographer has access to the previous radiographs and exposure factors, it generally is best to use the recommended exposure factors for the anatomic area and adjust the exposure techniques accordingly for any subsequent density error.

Anode Heel Effect

As a result of the angle of the x-ray tube's anode, the intensity along the longitudinal axis of the primary x-ray beam varies; this variance is called the *anode heel effect*. The **anode heel effect** is a decrease in the primary x-ray beam intensity on the anode side of the tube, making the primary beam on the cathode side of the tube more intense in comparison. Under certain circumstances, this decrease in intensity at the anode end of the primary beam could affect the uniformity of densities produced and could be visible on the radiographic image.

The anode heel effect is more visible on radiographs that use a short SID and a large x-ray field size. When a short SID is used, the collimator must be opened farther to achieve a particular projected field size. Opening the collimator more in the cathode-anode axis exposes the film to a wider variation in primary beam intensity. Likewise, the anode heel effect is less obvious on radiographs that use a long SID and a small field size. When a long SID is used, the collimator is opened less to achieve a particular projected field size. Opening the collimator less in the cathode-anode axis exposes the film to less of a variation in the primary beam intensity. The visibility of the anode heel effect on a radiographic image depends on the SID used, the x-ray beam field size, and the anatomic area of interest (Box 4-3).

BOX 4-3 *Effective Use of the Anode Heel Effect*

To produce anteroposterior (AP) thoracic spine radiographs with relatively similar densities throughout all 12 vertebrae, the radiographer should position the patient so that the cathode side of the tube is over the inferior portion of the spine (abdomen) and the anode side of the tube is over the superior portion of the spine (chest). Likewise, for extremities, the cathode side of the tube should be positioned over the proximal end (thickest) of the extremity and the anode side of the tube should be positioned over the distal end (thinnest) of the extremity.

Placing the thickest part of the anatomic area under the cathode end of the x-ray beam will help decrease the visibility of the anode heel effect. Because the beam is more intense on the cathode side and less intense on the anode side, this technique generally produces a radiograph that is more uniform in density along the long axis of the image.

Reciprocity Law

The **reciprocity law** states that the density produced on the radiograph will be equal for any combination of milliamperage and exposure time, as long as the product of mAs is equal. This law will hold true for direct-exposure radiography (without intensifying screens). When intensifying screens are used to expose the film, reciprocity failure can occur when extreme exposure times are used. Exposure times of more than 10 s or less than 10 ms will not consistently produce the expected density for a given mAs. At these extreme exposure times, the intensifying screen light emission may not produce equivalent exposure of the film. The radiographer must use caution when operating at or below 10 ms. The density produced at this low exposure time may not be equal to the density produced at a higher exposure time and lower milliamperage station combination. It is recommended that the radiographer select a reasonably low milliamperage to keep the exposure time to more than 10 ms so that sufficient density is produced.

Generator Output

Exposure techniques are developed in a radiographic room, depending on the type of generator used. Generators with more efficient output, such as three-phase units, require lower technique settings to produce an image comparable to those of single-phase units. The radiographer must be aware of the generator output when using different types of equipment, especially when performing examinations in different departments.

In addition, generator output variability can unexpectedly affect radiographic densities. X-ray generators must be calibrated periodically to ensure that they are producing consistent radiation output. Generator output variability is a quality control issue.

Tube Filtration

Small variation in the amount of tube filtration should not have any visible effect on the radiographic density. Variability of the x-ray tube filtration should be checked as a part of routine quality control checks on the radiographic equipment. X-ray tubes that have excessive or insufficient filtration may begin to affect the radiographic density. See Chapter 2 for a more thorough discussion of tube filtration.

Film Processing

Processing of the film after exposure to radiation has a major effect on both the density and the contrast of the radiograph. Variability of the processor in temperature, chemistry, or film transport can adversely affect the radiographic density or contrast. A more thorough discussion of processing and its effect on exposed film can be found in Chapter 7.

RADIOGRAPHIC CONTRAST

Radiographic contrast is a photographic factor that also affects the visibility of recorded detail. Contrast is the degree of difference between adjacent densities. The ability to distinguish between densities enables differences in anatomic tissues to be visualized. An image that has sufficient density but no differences in densities would appear as a homogeneous object (Figure 4-9). This appearance would indicate that the absorption characteristics of the object are equal. When the absorption characteristics of an object differ, the image presents with varying densities (Figure 4-10). In tissues in which the absorption characteristics differ, visualization of recorded detail is optimal when contrast is maximized.

Radiographic contrast can be described as high or low. A radiograph with few densities but great differences among them is said to have **high contrast.** This is also described as **short-scale contrast** (Figure 4-11). A radiograph with a large number of densities but little differences among them is said to have **low contrast.** This is also described as **long-scale contrast** (Figure 4-12).

Radiographic contrast is the combined result of two categories: **film (image receptor) contrast** and **subject contrast** (Box 4-4). Film, or image receptor, contrast is a result of the inherent properties manufactured into the type of film and how it is radiographed (direct exposure or with intensifying screens), along with the processing conditions. Subject contrast is a result of the absorption characteristics of the anatomic tissue radiographed and the level of kilovoltage used.

FIGURE 4-9 Radiograph of a homogeneous object having no differences in densities.

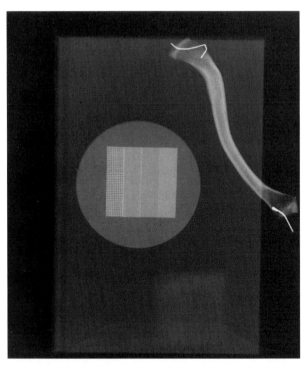

FIGURE 4-10 An object with different absorption characteristics produces an image with varying densities.

BOX 4-4 *Factors in Radiographic Contrast*

Subject Contrast	**Film (Image Receptor) Contrast**
Kilovoltage	Film type
Tissue composition	Direct exposure or intensifying screens
Contrast medium	Processing conditions

Unlike density, contrast is a more complex photographic factor. Evaluating radiographic quality in terms of contrast is more subjective (it is affected by individual preferences). In addition, specifying what level of radiographic contrast is optimal is difficult. The level of radiographic contrast desired in an image is determined by the composition of the anatomic tissue to be radiographed and the amount of information needed to visualize the tissue to make an accurate diagnosis. For example, the level of contrast desired in a chest radiograph is different from that required in a

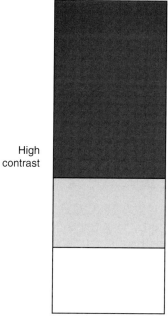

FIGURE 4-11 High-contrast (short-scale) image showing fewer gray tones and greater differences between individual densities.

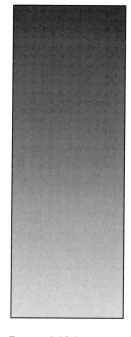

FIGURE 4-12 Low-contrast (long-scale) image showing many gray tones and little difference between individual densities.

radiograph of an extremity. Also, the composition of the anatomic area varies greatly between the chest and an extremity.

The radiographer must evaluate the composition of the anatomic structure to be radiographed and determine the factors that must be manipulated to produce the desired level of radiographic contrast. Achieving the desired level of contrast will maximize the amount of information visible to make a diagnosis. As with density, the ability to produce the desired level of radiographic contrast depends on the radiographer's knowledge about the controlling and influencing factors and on his or her clinical experience.

Radiographic contrast can be evaluated best when the radiographic density is adequate to visualize the density differences. When density is either too light or too dark, radiographic contrast cannot be assessed adequately. Therefore the following discussion focuses on factors that influence contrast, assuming radiographic density is adequate. This complex relationship between density and contrast is discussed in more detail in Chapter 8.

Factors that directly affect contrast are identified as controlling factors, whereas influencing factors indirectly affect contrast (Box 4-5).

Box 4-5 *Contrast*

Controlling Factor
Kilovoltage

Influencing Factors
Grids
Collimation
Object-to-image receptor distance
Anatomic part
Contrast media
Processing

Controlling Factor

Kilovoltage is considered the controlling factor for radiographic contrast (Box 4-6). The quality or penetrating power of the x-ray beam has the most direct effect on controlling the desired level of contrast.

Box 4-6 *Controlling Factor for Radiographic Contrast*

The kilovoltage or penetrating power of the x-ray beam controls the desired level of radiographic contrast.

Altering the penetrating power of the x-ray beam affects its absorption and transmission through the anatomic tissue being radiographed. High kilovoltage increases the penetrating power of the x-ray beam and results in lower absorption, more transmission, and fewer density differences in the anatomic tissues; this is described as low contrast (Figure 4-13). When a low kilovoltage is used, the x-ray beam penetration is decreased, resulting in more absorption, less transmission, and more density differences in the tissues; this is described as high contrast (Figure 4-14).

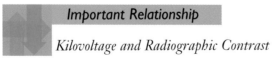

Important Relationship

Kilovoltage and Radiographic Contrast

High kilovoltage creates more densities but with fewer differences, resulting in a low-contrast (long-scale) image. Low kilovoltage creates fewer densities but with greater differences, resulting in a high-contrast (short-scale) image.

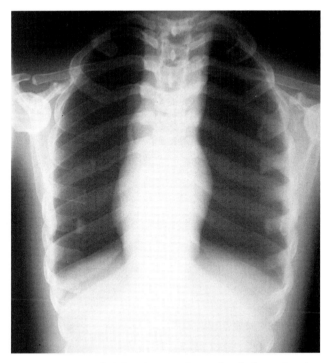

Figure 4-13 High-kilovoltage radiograph of chest showing low contrast.

The kilovoltage also affects the amount of scatter that occurs during the interaction of the x-ray beam and the anatomic tissue. A higher kilovoltage increases the amount of scatter radiation that could interact with the image receptor. Scatter radiation provides no useful information and only adds unwanted density, or fog, on the radiograph. Increasing the amount of fog on a radiograph always decreases the radiographic contrast.

Important Relationship

Kilovoltage, Scatter Radiation, and Radiographic Contrast

Increasing kilovoltage increases the amount of scatter radiation produced and decreases radiographic contrast. Decreasing the kilovoltage decreases scatter production and reduces the amount of fog, therefore increasing radiographic contrast.

The level of radiographic contrast desired, and therefore the kVp level selected, in an image depends on the type and composition of the anatomic tissue, the structures

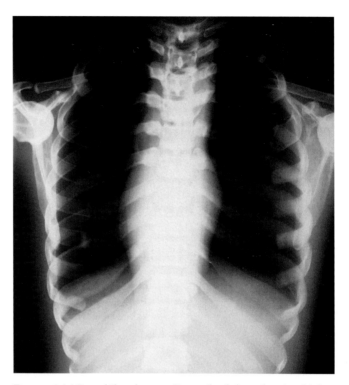

FIGURE 4-14 Low-kilovoltage radiograph of chest showing higher contrast than that in Figure 4-13.

that must be visualized, and to some extent, the diagnostician's preference. These factors make achieving a desired level of radiographic contrast more complex than achieving a desired level of radiographic density.

For most anatomic regions, there is an accepted range of kilovoltage that will provide an appropriate level of radiographic contrast. As long as the kilovoltage selected is sufficient to penetrate the anatomic part, the kVp can be further manipulated to alter the radiographic contrast.

Unlike density errors, radiographs generally are not repeated because of contrast errors. More often, the radiographer evaluates the level of contrast achieved and problem solves, if necessary, to improve upon the contrast for further radiographs or under similar circumstances that arise with a different patient.

If a repeat radiograph is necessary and kilovoltage is to be adjusted to either increase or decrease the level of contrast, the 15% rule provides an acceptable method of adjustment. In addition, to maintain the same density, whenever a 15% change is made in kVp, the radiographer must adjust the mAs by a factor of 2. Remember that a 15% change in kilovoltage will not produce the same effect across the entire range of kilovoltage used in radiography. A greater increase will be needed for high kilovoltage (90 and above) than for low kilovoltage (below 70).

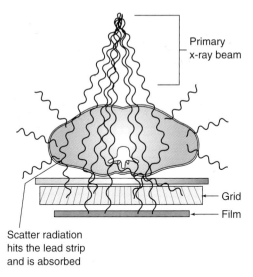

Primary
x-ray beam

Grid

Film

Scatter radiation
hits the lead strip
and is absorbed

FIGURE 4-15 Much of the scatter radiation toward the image receptor will be absorbed when a grid is used.

Influencing Factors

Most of the influencing factors affect radiographic contrast by controlling the amount of scatter radiation that reaches the image receptor. Limiting the amount of scatter radiation that reaches the image receptor always increases the radiographic contrast.

Grids

Radiographic grids affect contrast as a result of their absorption of the scatter radiation that exits the patient. A grid is placed between the patient and the image receptor. Much of the scatter radiation exiting the patient will not reach the image receptor when absorbed by a grid (Figure 4-15). The effect of less scatter, or unwanted density (fog), on the image is to increase the radiographic contrast. The more efficient a grid in absorbing scatter, the greater its effect on radiographic contrast. Grid construction and efficiency are discussed in greater detail in Chapter 5.

Collimation

Changes in the size of the x-ray field affect the amount of the tissue irradiated. A wider field size (less collimation) irradiates more tissue and causes more scatter radiation to be produced. The increased amount of scatter radiation reaching the image receptor results in less radiographic contrast. A smaller field size (more collimation) irradiates less tissue and reduces the amount of scatter radiation produced. The decreased amount of scatter radiation reaching the image receptor results in greater radiographic contrast.

Object-to-Image Receptor Distance

When sufficient distance between the object and image receptor exists, an air gap is created, causing the scatter radiation to miss the image receptor (Figure 4-16). Whenever the amount of scatter radiation reaching the image receptor is reduced, the radiographic contrast will be increased.

The exact amount of object-to-image receptor distance (OID) needed to increase contrast has not been specified. The amount of OID it takes to increase contrast partly depends on the percentage of scatter radiation exiting the patient. For anatomic areas that produce a high percentage of scatter radiation, less OID is needed to improve contrast than for anatomic areas that produce less scatter. In addition, because increased OID also decreases density, the change in contrast may be difficult to perceive.

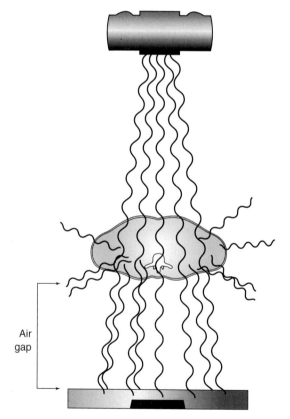

Air gap

FIGURE 4-16 A distance created between the object and image receptor will reduce the amount of scatter radiation reaching film.

Important Relationship

Scatter Radiation and Radiographic Contrast

Whenever the amount of scatter radiation reaching the image receptor is reduced, the radiographic contrast is increased (higher contrast).

Anatomic Part

The amount of radiographic contrast achieved is also influenced by the anatomic part to be radiographed. As mentioned earlier, subject contrast is one of the categories of radiographic contrast. The composition and thickness of the tissue and cell compactness affect its absorption characteristics. The absorption characteristics of the anatomic tissue will create the range of densities (contrast) produced on a radiograph. Tissues that have a higher atomic number will absorb more radiation than those with a lower atomic number.

Anatomic structures that have a wide range of tissue composition will demonstrate high subject contrast (Figure 4-17). In contrast, anatomic structures that consist of similar type tissue will demonstrate low subject contrast (Figure 4-18). The

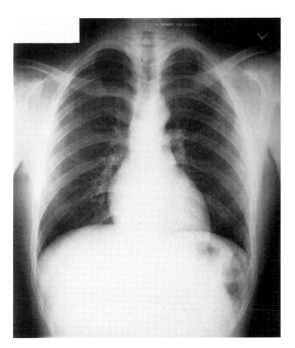

FIGURE 4-17 The chest is an anatomic area of high subject contrast because there is great variation in tissue composition.

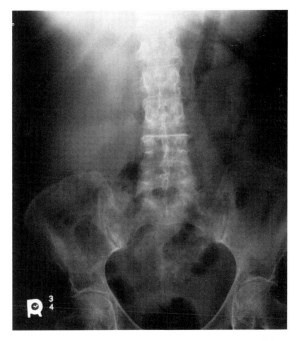

FIGURE 4-18 The abdomen is an anatomic area of low subject contrast because it is made up of similar tissue types.

radiographer cannot control the composition of the anatomic part to be radiographed. Changing the kilovoltage will alter the absorption characteristics of the tissues irradiated. Knowledge about the absorption characteristics of anatomic tissues combined with the effect of kilovoltage will aid the radiographer in producing a desired level of radiographic contrast.

For a given type of anatomic tissue, when the thickness is increased, the amount of scatter radiation is also increased and radiographic contrast decreased. Using a higher kilovoltage for a thicker part only adds to the increase in scatter radiation. Increased scatter radiation will continue to degrade the quality of the image because it creates fog, which decreases the contrast.

Contrast Media

A **contrast medium** (also called *contrast agent*) is used when imaging anatomic tissues that have low subject contrast. A contrast medium is a substance that can be instilled into the body by injection or ingestion. The type of contrast media used will change the absorption characteristics of the tissues by either increasing or decreasing the attenuation of the x-ray beam. Positive contrast agents, such as barium and iodine, have a high

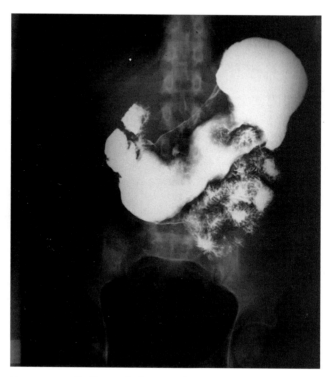

FIGURE 4-19 Radiograph showing decreased density because of the increase in x-ray beam attenuation by use of a positive contrast media agent.

atomic number and absorb more x-rays (increase attenuation) than the surrounding tissue (Figure 4-19). Negative contrast agents, such as air, decrease the attenuation of the x-ray beam and transmit more radiation than the surrounding tissue (Figure 4-20). Positive contrast agents produce less radiographic density than the adjacent tissues. Negative contrast agents produce more radiographic density than the adjacent tissues.

The use of a contrast agent is an effective method of increasing the radiographic contrast when radiographing areas of low subject contrast. Box 4-7 summarizes the photographic factors that control and influence the visibility of recorded detail.

Box 4-7 *Photographic Factors That Control and Influence the Visibility of Recorded Detail*

Anatomic part	Film-screen system speed
Anode heel effect	Generator output
Collimation	Grids
Contrast media	Kilovoltage
Distance	Milliamperage
Exposure time	Reciprocity law
Film processing	Tube filtration

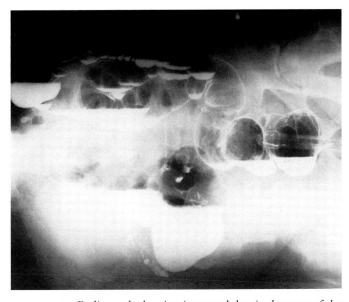

FIGURE 4-20 Radiograph showing increased density because of the decrease in x-ray beam attenuation by use of a negative contrast media agent.

As mentioned previously, the quality of a radiographic image depends on both the visibility and the sharpness of the recorded detail. Adequate visualization of the anatomic area of interest is just one component of radiographic quality. The ability to visualize an unsharp image is not sufficient for an image of diagnostic quality. The level of sharpness of the recorded image will determine the geometric properties of the radiograph.

Geometric Properties (Sharpness)

The **geometric properties** of an image refer to the sharpness of structural lines recorded in the radiographic image. A radiographic image cannot be an exact reconstruction of the anatomic structure. Some information is always lost during the process of image formation. It is the radiographer's responsibility to minimize the amount of information lost by accurately manipulating the factors that affect the sharpness of the recorded image. Optimal geometric quality is achieved by maximizing the amount of recorded detail and minimizing the amount of image distortion (Figure 4-21).

RECORDED DETAIL

Recorded detail refers to the distinctness or sharpness of the structural lines that make up the recorded image. The ability of a radiographic image to demonstrate sharp lines will determine the quality of the recorded detail. The imaging process makes it impossible to produce a radiographic image without some degree of unsharpness. A radiographic image that has a large amount of recorded detail will minimize the amount of unsharpness of the anatomic structural lines. The quality of the recorded detail is controlled by minimizing geometric unsharpness and receptor unsharpness and by eliminating motion unsharpness.

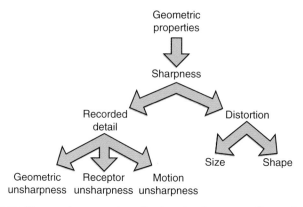

FIGURE 4-21 Geometric properties affecting the sharpness of recorded detail.

Geometric Unsharpness

The amount of **geometric unsharpness** is a result of the relationship among the size of the focal spot, SID, and OID (Figure 4-22). Manipulating each variable individually or in combination will alter the amount of unsharpness recorded in the image.

Focal Spot Size

The physical dimensions of the focal spot on the anode target in x-ray tubes used in standard radiographic applications usually range from 0.5 to 1.2 mm. Focal spot size is determined by the filament size. When the radiographer selects a particular focal spot size, he or she is actually selecting a filament size that will be energized during x-ray production. The radiographer can select on the control panel whether to use a small focal spot size or a large one. Small focal spot sizes are usually 0.5 or 0.6 mm in size, and large focal spot sizes are usually 1.0 or 1.2 mm in size. Focal spot size is an important consideration for the radiographer to make because focal spot size controls recorded detail (Figure 4-23).

Important Relationship

Focal Spot Size and Recorded Detail

As focal spot size increases, unsharpness increases and recorded detail decreases; as focal spot size decreases, unsharpness decreases and recorded detail increases.

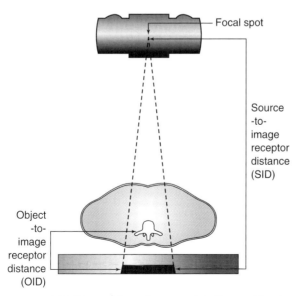

FIGURE 4-22 Geometric unsharpness is influenced by the relationship among focal spot, SID, and OID.

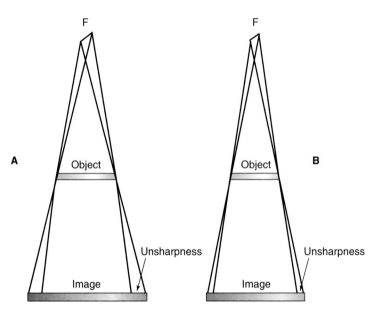

FIGURE 4-23 Focal spot size influences the amount of unsharpness recorded in the image. As focal spot size changes, so does the amount of unsharpness. **A,** Larger focal spot. **B,** Smaller focal spot.

In general, the smallest focal spot size available should be used for every exposure. Unfortunately, exposure is limited with a small focal spot size. When a small focal spot is used, the heat created during the exposure is concentrated to a smaller area and could cause tube damage. The radiographer must weigh the importance of improved recorded detail for a particular examination or anatomic part to the amount of exposure used. Modern radiographic x-ray generators are equipped with safety circuits that will prevent an exposure from being made if that exposure will exceed the tube loading capacity for the focal spot size selected. Repeated exposures just under the limitation made over a long period can still jeopardize the life of the x-ray tube.

 Practical Tip

Selecting Focal Spot Size

The radiographer should select the smallest focal spot size, considering the amount of x-ray exposure used and the amount of recorded detail required for the radiographic examination.

Distance

As discussed previously in this chapter, distance plays an important role in radiographic imaging. Just as the intensity of the x-ray beam is altered when changing the distance between the source and object or the object and receptor, so is the amount of unsharpness recorded on the image. Because of the diverging properties of the x-ray beam, a geometric relationship exists among the source of x-rays, the object, and image receptor (Figure 4-24).

Figure 4-25 demonstrates that when the SID is increased, the amount of edge unsharpness is decreased. As the distance between the source and image receptor increases, the diverging x-rays become more perpendicular to the object radiographed.

Important Relationship

SID, Unsharpness, and Recorded Detail

Increasing the SID decreases the amount of unsharpness and increases the amount of recorded detail in the image, whereas decreasing the SID increases the amount of unsharpness and decreases the recorded detail.

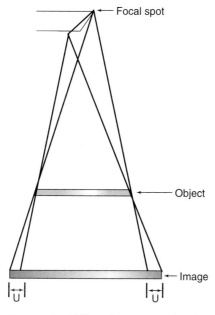

FIGURE 4-24 There is a geometric relationship among the x-ray source, object, and image receptor. *U,* Unsharpness.

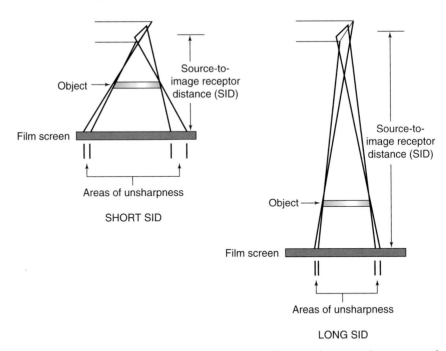

FIGURE 4-25 Increasing source-to-image receptor distance decreases the amount of edge (geometric) unsharpness.

Standard distances for SID are used in radiography to accommodate equipment limitations. Except for chest and cervical spine radiography, a 40-inch (100-cm) or 48-inch (122-cm) SID is the standard used in radiography.

In addition to SID, the OID also affects the amount of unsharpness recorded on the image. Optimal recorded detail is achieved when the OID is zero. Unfortunately, this cannot realistically be achieved in radiographic imaging.

As the exit beam leaves the patient, it continues to diverge. When distance is created between the area of interest and the image receptor, the diverging exit beam records edge unsharpness within the image (Figure 4-26).

Important Relationship

OID, Unsharpness, and Recorded Detail

Increasing the OID increases the amount of unsharpness and decreases the recorded detail, whereas decreasing the amount of OID decreases the amount of unsharpness and increases the recorded detail.

The distance between the area of interest and the image receptor has the greatest effect on the amount of geometric unsharpness recorded. When possible, the distance

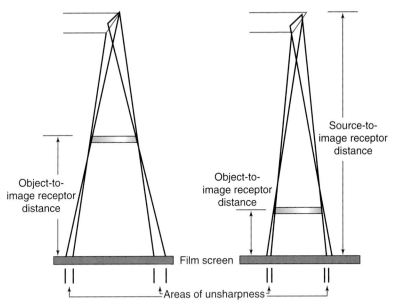

Film screen

Areas of unsharpness

Source-to-image receptor distance

Object-to-image receptor distance

FIGURE 4-26 Increasing object-to-image receptor distance increases the amount of edge (geometric) unsharpness.

between the area of interest and the image receptor should be kept to a minimum. When a film-screen image receptor is used and placed in a table Bucky, some amount of increased OID will always occur. It is the radiographer's responsibility to position the area of interest as close to the image receptor as possible to minimize the amount of unsharpness recorded.

The relationship among the variables of focal spot size and distance can be demonstrated mathematically by the geometric unsharpness formula (Box 4-8).

Box 4-8 *Geometric Unsharpness Formula*

$$\text{Geometric unsharpness} = \frac{\text{Focal spot size} \times \text{OID}}{\text{SOD}}$$

where

Focal spot size = Dimensions of the effective focal spot in millimeters (mm)
OID = The distance between the object (area of interest) and the image receptor
SOD = The distance between the focal spot (source) and object (area of interest)
SOD = SID − OID

When calculating the amount of geometric unsharpness, the radiographer must keep the distance measurement in the same units (i.e., inches or centimeters). This will cancel the units out and result in the geometric unsharpness unit of millimeters.

The unit of geometric unsharpness provides a method of mathematically comparing the amount of unsharpness present for a given focal spot size and distance.

X *Mathematical Application*

Calculating Geometric Unsharpness

The amount of geometric unsharpness can be calculated for each of the following images to determine which image has increased geometric unsharpness.

Image 1	**Image 2**
Focal spot size = 0.6 mm	Focal spot size = 1.2 mm
SID = 40 inches	SID = 56 inches
OID = 0.25 inch	OID = 4.0 inches

Image 1

$$\frac{0.6 \text{ mm} \times 0.25 \text{ inch}}{39.75 \text{ inches}} ; \frac{0.15}{39.75}$$

Image 2

$$\frac{1.2 \text{ mm} \times 4 \text{ inches}}{52 \text{ inches}} ; \frac{4.8}{52}$$

Geometric unsharpness of Image 1 = 0.004 mm
Geometric unsharpness of Image 2 = 0.09 mm

Image 2 has the greatest amount of unsharpness.

Although minimizing geometric unsharpness is important, the radiographer also must consider the effect of these variables on the x-ray tube. The smallest focal spot size may not be the best choice when radiographing the lateral lumbar spine, nor is the amount of recorded detail as important in this anatomic region when compared with extremities. In addition, using a 72-inch SID is not practical for most radiographic studies, although it is justified when imaging the chest or lateral cervical spine.

Practical Tip

Minimizing Geometric Unsharpness

The radiographer should select the smallest focal spot size when maximal recorded detail is important; he or she should also consider the amount of heat load within the x-ray tube. In addition, the radiographer should select the standard SID when OID is minimal. When increased OID is unavoidable, the SID should be increased slightly to compensate.

The radiographer has the most control over the amount of unsharpness recorded in the image by manipulating the focal spot size, selecting the appropriate SID, and maintaining minimal OID.

Image Receptor Unsharpness

The type of device used to record the image also affects the amount of unsharpness recorded in the image. In conventional radiography, differing intensifying screen-film combinations have created a complex system of image receptors. Variations in the construction and composition of the intensifying screen combined with different types of radiographic film affect not only the photographic properties of the image but also its geometric properties.

One of the significant advancements in image receptors has been their ability to limit the amount of x-rays needed to produce a visible image. The ability to reduce the exposure to the patient has been at a cost to the quality of the image, mostly in recorded detail.

As mentioned in the section on film-screen systems' effect on density, the higher the relative speed of the film-screen system, the fewer x-rays needed to create the image. The changes that are needed to increase the relative speed of the film-screen system will also decrease the amount of recorded detail within the radiographic image. The composition and construction of intensifying film-screen systems are discussed in more detail in Chapter 6.

Important Relationship

Intensifying Film-Screen Speed, Recorded Detail, and Unsharpness

Increasing the relative speed of the intensifying film-screen system decreases the recorded detail and increases the amount of unsharpness recorded in the image. Decreasing the relative speed of the intensifying film-screen system increases the recorded detail and decreases the amount of unsharpness recorded in the image.

Because the radiographic film normally is placed between two intensifying screens, any distance that is created between the film and screen will cause increased unsharpness to be recorded in the image. Poor film-screen contact creates an area of unsharpness because the light emitted from the intensifying screen phosphor crystal diverges from its origin. When there is distance between the film and phosphor crystal, the light spread causes unsharp structural lines to be recorded in the image (Figure 4-27). It is important to maintain good film-screen contact to maximize recorded detail. If good film-screen contact cannot be maintained, the screen must be repaired or discarded.

Measuring Recorded Detail

Recorded detail can be measured and is expressed as resolution. **Resolution** is the ability of the imaging system to resolve or distinguish between two adjacent structures. Resolution can be expressed in the unit of line pairs per millimeter (Lp/mm) (Figure 4-28). A resolution grid is a device used to record and measure line pairs. The greater the number of line pairs per millimeter resolved, the greater the resolution and therefore recorded detail. In the space of 1 mm, the number of line pairs resolved will determine the quality of the recorded detail. Each line pair is made up of a line and a space. Visual acuity of the human eye is limited to the ability to discern 5 Lp/mm. At this level, each line measures 0.1 mm and a line pair measures 0.2 mm. An imaging system that can resolve a greater number of line pairs within 1 mm (e.g., 8 to 10 Lp/mm) is said to have improved recorded detail. The average human eye would not be able to distinguish this improved recorded detail. However, when resolution is measured below 5 Lp/mm (e.g., 2 to 3 Lp/mm), the reduced recorded detail can be visualized.

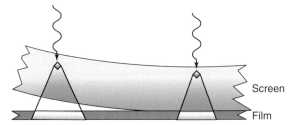

Screen
Film

FIGURE 4-27 Poor film-screen contact will cause increased unsharpness.

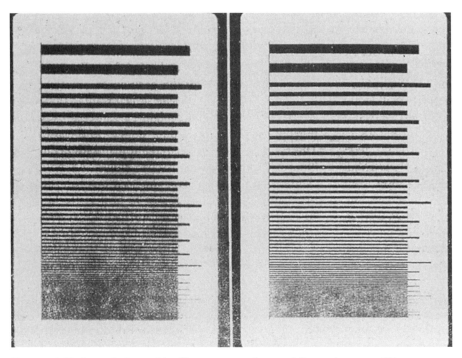

FIGURE 4-28 A resolution grid will measure and record line pairs per millimeter. *From Mosby's instructional radiographic series: radiographic imaging, St Louis, 1998, Mosby.*

Motion Unsharpness

Motion unsharpness has the most detrimental effect on the recorded detail of the radiographic image. Motion of the tube, part, or image receptor causes a profound decrease in recorded detail (Figure 4-29). Motion must not just be decreased, it must be eliminated.

Important Relationship

Motion and Recorded Detail

Motion of the tube, patient or part, or image receptor greatly decreases recorded detail.

Unsharpness resulting from patient motion, known as **blur,** is the most detrimental factor to good recorded detail. Unsharpness resulting from patient motion can be classified as voluntary (within the patient's control) or involuntary (outside of patient's control, such as peristalsis). Most motion on radiographs results from the patient moving during the exposure. The radiographer can control patient motion to

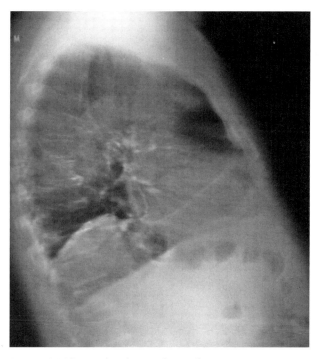

FIGURE 4-29 Image showing motion unsharpness. *From* Mosby's instructional radiographic series: radiographic imaging, *St Louis, 1998, Mosby.*

some degree. Patients who are least likely to cooperate, and therefore move, are pediatric patients, those with conditions such as Parkinson's disease that cause involuntary shaking, and those who are otherwise unwilling or unable to cooperate, such as intoxicated and traumatized patients.

Practical Tip

Eliminating Motion

Patient motion can be controlled by the radiographer by doing the following:

1. Using short exposure times compensated for by higher mA
2. Communicating good instructions for the patient to assist in immobilization
3. Using physical immobilization, such as sandbags, tape, or other devices, as deemed necessary

If a patient needs to be physically held, it is generally recommended that the holder not be a person who routinely is exposed to x-rays. The holder should always wear lead shielding and, if female, be evaluated for the possibility of pregnancy before making the exposure.

A less typical type of motion unsharpness can be caused by equipment, such as undesirable motion of the tube, table, or image receptor. Motion of the tube or image receptor is not very likely because tube assemblies and film trays have locks that are easily used by the radiographer.

DISTORTION

Distortion results from the radiographic misrepresentation of either the size (magnification) or shape of the anatomic part. When the image is distorted, recorded detail is also reduced.

Size Distortion (Magnification)

The term **size distortion/magnification** refers to an increase in the object's image size compared with its true, or actual, size. Radiographic images of objects are always magnified in terms of the true object size. The distances (SID and OID) used play an important role in minimizing the amount of size distortion of the radiographic image.

Object-to-Image Receptor Distance

Magnification of the true object will occur because there is always some OID during radiography. OID has a direct relationship with magnification.

As OID increases, size distortion (magnification) increases; as OID decreases, size distortion (magnification) decreases.

Because radiographers produce radiographs of three-dimensional objects, some size distortion always occurs as a result of OID. Even if the object is in close contact with the image receptor, some part of the object will be farther away from the image receptor than other parts of the object. Those parts of the object that are farther away from the image receptor will be demonstrated radiographically with more size distortion than parts of the object that are closer to the image receptor.

Figure 4-30 shows how two objects of the same size are demonstrated radiographically using a short OID and a long OID. Notice how a long OID produces more size distortion than a short OID does.

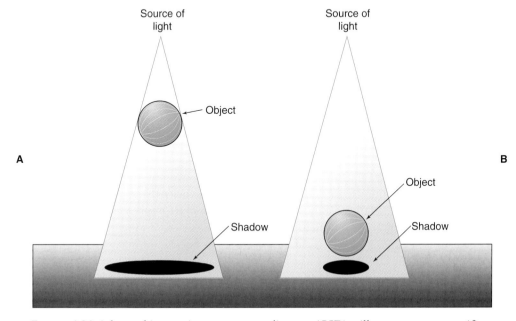

FIGURE 4-30 A long object-to-image receptor distance (OID) will create more magnification than a short OID. The shadow in **A** is larger than that in **B** because the object is farther from the image receptor.

Practical Tip

Minimizing OID

The radiographer should always try to minimize OID as much as possible to reduce size distortion (magnification). Within the protocol of the examination, it is always best to try to position the area of interest closest to the image receptor to minimize size distortion of that area.

Source-to-Image Receptor Distance

SID also influences the total amount of size distortion represented on a radiograph. Although OID has the greatest effect on size distortion, SID is still an important factor for the radiographer to control to minimize size distortion. SID and magnification have an inverse relationship.

Important Relationship

SID and Size Distortion

As SID increases, size distortion (magnification) decreases; as SID decreases, size distortion (magnification) increases.

Figure 4-31 illustrates how a long SID produces less size distortion than a short SID does. In some situations it is difficult to minimize OID because of factors or conditions outside of the radiographer's control. In these instances size distortion can still be reduced by increasing SID.

Calculating Magnification

To observe the effect of geometric factors on size distortion, it is necessary to consider the magnification factor. The **magnification factor (MF)** indicates how much size distortion or magnification is demonstrated on a radiograph. The MF can be expressed mathematically by the following formula:

$$MF = \frac{SID}{SOD}$$

SOD represents **source-to-object distance,** which refers to the distance from the x-ray source (focal spot) to the object being radiographed. SOD can be expressed mathematically as follows:

$$SOD = SID - OID$$

SOD is also demonstrated in Figure 4-32.

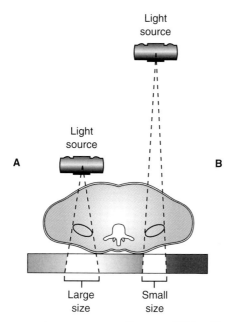

FIGURE 4-31 A long source-to-image receptor distance (SID) will create less magnification than a short SID. The shadow in **A** is bigger than that in **B** because the object is closer to the light source. The same happens with radiographic images.

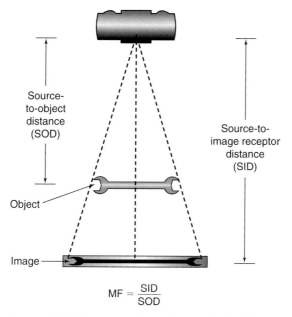

$$MF = \frac{SID}{SOD}$$

FIGURE 4-32 Source-to-object distance is the distance between the source of x-ray and the object radiographed.

An MF of 1.00 indicates no magnification. No magnification means that the size of the radiographic image matches the true object size. This is an impossible situation because some magnification exists on every radiograph. An MF greater than 1.0 can be expressed as a percentage of magnification.

X Mathematical Application

The Magnification Factor

A posteroanterior (PA) projection of the chest was produced with an SID of 72 inches and an OID of 3 inches. What is the MF?

$$MF = \frac{72 \text{ inches}}{69 \text{ inches}}$$

$$MF = 1.044$$

In the case of the Mathematical Application for MF, an MF of 1.044 means that the image is 4.4% larger than the true object size. It should be noted that the MF computed here is a minimum. A 3-inch OID implies that the anterior surface of the patients chest was 3 inches away from the image receptor for a PA projection. Anatomy that is posterior to the anterior chest wall is farther away from the image receptor and will be magnified even more.

Once the MF is known, the object size can then be determined. This requires the use of another formula:

$$\text{Object size} = \frac{\text{Image size}}{\text{MF}}$$

It may be helpful to know the measurement of the true object size in comparison to its size on a radiographic image.

X Mathematical Application

Determining Object Size

On a PA chest film taken with an SID of 72 inches and an OID of 3 inches (SOD is equal to 69 inches), the size of a round lesion in the right lung measures 1.5 inches in diameter on the radiograph. The MF has been determined to be 1.044. What is the object size of this lesion?

$$\text{Object size} = \frac{1.5 \text{ inches}}{1.044}$$

$$\text{Object size} = 1.44 \text{ inches}$$

Perhaps the most practical use of these formulas is to observe how changing the SID and OID affects the true object size. Size distortion or magnification can be increased by decreasing the SID or by increasing the OID. This increase in magnification can be demonstrated mathematically by using the MF and then calculating the change in the true size of the object on the radiographic image.

Shape Distortion

In addition to size distortion, objects that are being imaged can also be misrepresented radiographically by distortion of their shape. Shape distortion can appear in two different ways radiographically: as elongation or as foreshortening. **Elongation** refers to images of objects that appear longer than the true object. **Foreshortening** refers to images that appear shorter than the true objects. Examples of elongation and foreshortening can be seen in Figure 4-33.

Shape distortion can occur with inaccurate central ray (CR) alignment of the tube, the part being radiographed, or the image receptor. Any misalignment of the CR among these three factors—tube, part, or image receptor—will alter the shape of the part recorded on the film. In addition, shape distortion becomes more

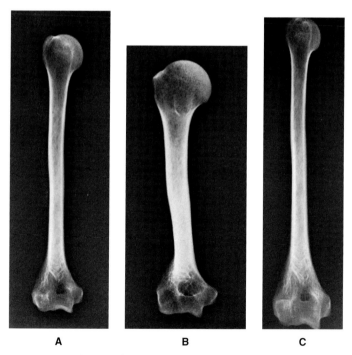

| A | B | C |

FIGURE 4-33 A, No distortion. **B,** Foreshortened. **C,** Elongated.
From Mosby's instructional radiographic series: radiographic imaging, *St Louis, 1998, Mosby.*

obvious if the CR of the primary beam is not directed to enter or exit the anatomy as required for the particular projection or position (off centering). This happens because the path of individual photons in the primary beam become more divergent as the distance increases from the CR. The radiographer must properly control alignment of the tube, part, and image receptor, and he or she must properly direct the CR to minimize shape distortion.

Sometimes, shape distortion is used to an advantage in particular projections or positions. CR angulation, for example, is sometimes required to elongate a part so that a particular anatomic structure can be visualized better. Also, CR angulation is sometimes required to eliminate superimposition of objects that normally would obstruct visualization of the area of interest. In general, shape distortion is not a necessary or desirable characteristic of radiographs.

Practical Tip

Minimizing Shape Distortion

Elongation and foreshortening can be minimized by ensuring the proper CR alignment of the following:

1. X-ray tube
2. Part
3. Image receptor
4. Entry or exit point of the CR

The quality of the radiographic image depends on a multitude of variables. Knowledge of these variables and their radiographic effect will assist the radiographer in producing quality radiographs. Table 4-2 provides a chart demonstrating the radiographic effects of the variables discussed in this chapter.

TABLE 4-2   **VARIABLES AND THEIR EFFECT ON BOTH THE PHOTOGRAPHIC AND GEOMETRIC PROPERTIES OF THE RADIOGRAPHIC IMAGE**

Radiographic Variables	Photographic Properties		Geometric Properties	
	Density	Contrast	Recorded Detail	Distortion
↑ mAs*	↑	0	0	0
↓ mAs	↓	0	0	0
↑ kVp	↑	↓	0	0
↓ kVp	↓	↑	0	0
↑ SID	↓	0	↑	↓
↓ SID	↑	0	↓	↑
↑ OID†	↓	↑	↓	↑
↓ OID	↑	↓	↑	↓
↑ Grid ratio	↓	↑	0	0
↓ Grid ratio	↑	↓	0	0
↑ Film-screen speed	↑	0	↓	0
↓ Film-screen speed	↓	0	↑	0
↑ Collimation	↓	↑	0	0
↓ Collimation	↑	↓	0	0
↑ Focal spot size	0	0	↓	0
↓ Focal spot size	0	0	↑	0
↑ Central ray angle	↓	0	↓	↑

mAs, The product of milliamperage and exposure time; *kVp*, kilovoltage peak; *SID*, source-to-image receptor distance; *OID*, object-to-image receptor distance; ↑, increased effect; ↓, decreased effect; *0*, no effect.
*The mAs has no significant effect on contrast as long as densities remain within diagnostic range.
†The amount of OID needed to affect contrast depends on the type of anatomic part being imaged.

F I L M   C R I T I Q U E

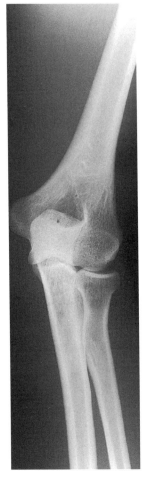 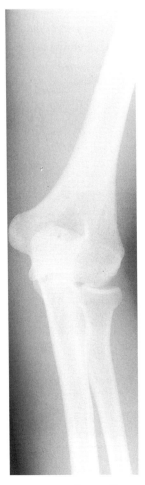 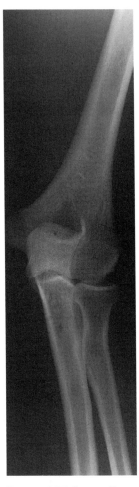 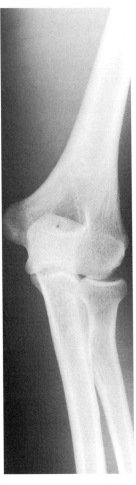

Figure 4-34 Image A was produced using 60 kVp, 100 mA at 0.040 s, 100 speed film-screen combination, 40-inch SID, and minimal OID.

Figure 4-35 Image B was produced using 60 kVp, 80 mA at 0.025 s, 100 speed film-screen combination, 40-inch SID, and minimal OID.

Figure 4-36 Image C was produced using 69 kVp, 160 mA at 0.025 s, 100 speed film-screen combination, 40-inch SID, and minimal OID.

Figure 4-37 Image D was produced using 60 kVp, 200 mA at 0.020 s, 100 speed film-screen combination, 40-inch SID, and 3-inch OID.

1. Given Image A is of optimal quality, discuss the quality of the other images.

2. For each image, evaluate its exposure variables and discuss their effect on the quality of the image (regardless of whether it is apparent on the radiograph).

3. For each image, identify any adjustments that could be made in the exposure factors to produce an image comparable to Image A.

Review Questions

1. A radiograph that needs no improvement is defined as
   A. unacceptable.
   B. optimal.
   C. inadequate.
   D. diagnostic.

2. Factors that affect the visibility of a radiographic image are known as
   A. resolution.
   B. geometric.
   C. densitometric.
   D. photographic.

3. A radiograph that has insufficient density would best be described as
   A. overexposed.
   B. overdeveloped.
   C. underexposed.
   D. underdeveloped.

4. Which of the following is equivalent to doubling the mAs?
   A. Halve the film-screen speed.
   B. Halve the OID.
   C. Double the SID.
   D. Increase kVp by 15%.

5. A radiograph was taken using 65 kVp, 200 mA at 0.10 s. The image needs to be repeated because it is too dark. What exposure technique adjustment would be best?
   A. 65 kVp, 200 mA at 0.05 s
   B. 86 kVp, 200 mA at 0.025 s
   C. 75 kVp, 200 mA at 0.20 s
   D. 55 kVp, 200 mA at 0.10 s

6. What is the relationship between milliamperage and exposure time to maintain density?
   A. Linear
   B. Inverse
   C. Proportional
   D. Direct

7. When repeating a radiograph to correct for a density error, it is recommended to adjust the mAs by a factor of
   A. $\frac{1}{2}$
   B. 2
   C. 3
   D. 4

8. Which of the following factors when *decreased* will *increase* density: 1.) grid ratio, 2.) focal spot size, or 3.) part thickness?
   A. 1 and 2 only
   B. 1 and 3 only
   C. 2 and 3 only
   D. 1, 2, and 3

9. How will radiographic density be affected when the SID is decreased by half?
   A. Increased
   B. Increased by half
   C. Decreased
   D. Decreased by half

10. A radiograph was produced using 85 kVp, 300 mA at 0.2 s. The density is sufficient, but the contrast is too low. Which of the following exposure technique changes would be best to increase the radiographic contrast?
    A. 98 kVp, 300 mA at 0.1 s
    B. 85 kVp, 300 mA at 0.4 s
    C. 72 kVp, 300 mA at 0.4 s
    D. 65 kVp, 300 mA at 0.2 s

11. A radiographic image described as having many shades of gray would be
    A. low density.
    B. low contrast.
    C. high density.
    D. high contrast.

12. The visible differences between adjacent radiographic densities defines
    A. fog.
    B. density.
    C. contrast.
    D. resolution.

13. Which of the following will increase radiographic contrast?
    A. Increasing part thickness
    B. Increasing the grid ratio
    C. Increasing the kilovoltage
    D. Increasing filtration

14. Radiographic contrast can be increased by
    A. increasing mAs.
    B. increasing kVp.
    C. decreasing grid ratio.
    D. adding contrast media.

15. What factor has the most direct effect on radiographic contrast?
    A. mAs
    B. SID
    C. Grids
    D. kVp

16. Recorded detail is defined as
    A. accuracy of structural lines recorded.
    B. visibility of the structural lines.
    C. misrepresentation of the shape of the structural lines.
    D. amount of structural lines.

17. The amount of unsharpness created using a focal spot of 0.6 mm, an SID of 36 inches, and an OID of 3 inches is
A. 0.005
B. 0.055
C. 0.567
D. 0.635

18. What is the image size of a part measuring 2.5 cm using an SID of 100 cm, an OID of 5 cm, and a focal spot of 1.25 mm?
A. 2.37 cm
B. 2.50 cm
C. 2.63 cm
D. 2.75 cm

19. Using a smaller focal spot size will have what effect on the radiographic image?
A. Increase density
B. Decrease contrast
C. Decrease distortion
D. Increase recorded detail

20. Shape distortion can be created by
A. angling the CR.
B. decreasing the SID.
C. increasing the focal spot size.
D. increasing the OID.

CHAPTER 5

Scatter Control

BEAM-RESTRICTING DEVICES

BEAM RESTRICTION AND SCATTER RADIATION

Collimation and Contrast
Compensating for Collimation

TYPES OF BEAM-RESTRICTING DEVICES

Aperture Diaphragms
Cones and Cylinders
Collimators
Automatic Collimators

RADIOGRAPHIC GRIDS

GRID CONSTRUCTION

Grid Pattern
Grid Focus

TYPES OF GRIDS

GRID PERFORMANCE

GRID CUTOFF

Types of Grid Cutoff
    Upside Down Focused
    Lateral Decentering
    Distance Decentering

MOVING GRIDS

Reciprocating Grids
Disadvantages

GRID USE

THE AIR GAP TECHNIQUE

FILM CRITIQUE

REVIEW QUESTIONS

Controlling the amount of scatter radiation that reaches the image receptor is essential in creating an optimal quality radiograph. Scatter radiation is detrimental to radiographic quality because it adds unwanted density to the radiograph without adding any patient information. Therefore the radiographer must try to minimize the amount of scatter radiation reaching the image receptor.

Beam-restricting devices and radiographic grids are tools the radiographer can use to limit the amount of scatter radiation reaching the image receptor. Beam-restricting devices decrease the amount of tissue irradiated, thereby reducing the amount of scatter radiation produced. Radiographic grids are used to improve the radiographic image quality by absorbing scatter radiation that exits the patient.

Beam-Restricting Devices

The unrestricted primary beam is cone shaped and projects a round field on the patient and image receptor (Figure 5-1). Image receptors can be rectangular or square

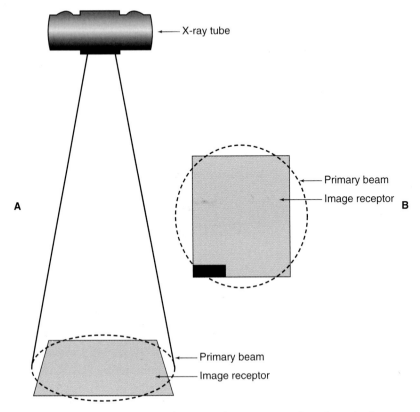

FIGURE 5-1 The unrestricted primary beam is cone shaped, projecting a circular field. **A,** Side view. **B,** View from above.

and therefore do not match the projected shape of the primary beam. If a radiographer does not restrict the beam, an increase in radiation exposure to the patient would occur because the primary beam would exceed the boundaries of the image receptor. The purpose of restricting the primary beam is to decrease the dose the patient receives by limiting the field of exposure. This is accomplished with a beam-restricting device. The terms **beam restriction** and **collimation** are used interchangeably; they refer to decreasing the size of the projected radiation field. The term *collimation* is probably used more often than the term *beam restriction* because collimators are the most popular type of beam-restricting device. Increasing collimation means decreasing field size, and decreasing collimation means increasing field size.

Important Relationship

Collimation and Patient Dose

As collimation increases, field size decreases; therefore patient dose also decreases. As collimation decreases, field size increases; therefore patient dose increases.

A **beam-restricting device** is extraneous to the x-ray tube housing and changes the shape and size of the primary beam. In addition to decreasing patient dose, beam-restricting devices also increase the quality of the image by reducing the amount of scatter radiation that the image receptor is exposed to, thereby increasing the radiographic contrast.

Important Relationship

Beam Restriction, Scatter Control, and Contrast

Beam restriction reduces the amount of scatter radiation produced, thus increasing radiographic contrast.

Beam Restriction and Scatter Radiation

Beam restriction is used to decrease patient dose by limiting the size and shape of the primary beam. Another benefit of using beam restriction is a reduction in the intensity of scatter radiation that is produced inside the patient during exposure. This reduction decreases the amount of scatter radiation that reaches the image receptor.

The relationship between collimation (field size) and intensity of scatter radiation is illustrated in Figure 5-2. As stated previously, collimation means decreasing the size of the projected field, so increasing collimation means decreasing field size, and decreasing collimation means increasing field size.

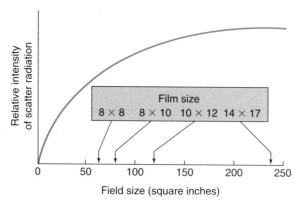

FIGURE 5-2 As field size increases, the relative intensity of scatter radiation increases.

Important Relationship

Collimation and Scatter Radiation

As collimation increases, the field size decreases and the intensity of scatter radiation decreases; as collimation decreases, the field size increases and the intensity of scatter radiation increases.

The term *intensity* is used in the statement of these two relationships to indicate quantity of scattered photons.

COLLIMATION AND CONTRAST

Because collimation decreases field size, less scatter radiation is produced inside the patient and on the radiographic tabletop. Thus less scatter radiation reaches the image receptor. As described in Chapter 4, this affects the radiographic contrast.

Important Relationship

Collimation and Radiographic Contrast

As collimation increases, radiographic contrast increases; as collimation decreases, radiographic contrast decreases.

COMPENSATING FOR COLLIMATION

An increase in collimation also affects radiographic density. Increasing collimation decreases the number of photons that strike the patient and image receptor and decreases the amount of scatter radiation produced. Therefore exposure factors may need to be changed when collimating.

TABLE 5-1	RESTRICTING THE PRIMARY BEAM
Increased Factor	**Result**
Collimation	Patient dose **decreases.**
	Scatter radiation **decreases.**
	Radiographic contrast **increases.**
	Radiographic density **decreases.**
Field size	Patient dose **increases.**

Important Relationship

Collimation and Radiographic Density

As collimation increases, radiographic density decreases; as collimation decreases, radiographic density increases.

Practical Tip

Compensating for Collimation

When collimating significantly (changing from a 11 × 14 inch field size to a small, 4-inch-diameter cone), the radiographer must increase exposure to compensate for the loss of density that will otherwise occur. The kilovoltage peak (kVp) value should not be increased. Increasing the kVp value will decrease contrast. To change density only, the product of milliamperage and exposure time (mAs) should be changed.

It has been recommended that significant collimation requires an increase in as much as 30% to 50% of the mAs to compensate for the loss in density that occurs because of collimation.

Important relationships regarding restricting the primary beam are summarized in Table 5-1.

Types of Beam-Restricting Devices

Several different types of beam-restricting devices are available; however, they differ in sophistication and utility. All beam-restricting devices are made of metal or a combination of metals that readily absorb x-rays.

APERTURE DIAPHRAGMS

The simplest type of beam-restricting device is the aperture diaphragm. An **aperture diaphragm** is a flat piece of lead (diaphragm) that has a hole (aperture) in it. Commercially made aperture diaphragms are available (Figure 5-3), as are those that are homemade (hospital-made) for purposes specific to a radiographic unit. Aperture diaphragms are easy to use. They slide into slots at the bottom of a collimator, or they can be taped directly onto the tube housing in the absence of a collimator. An aperture diaphragm can be made by cutting rubberized lead into the size needed to create the diaphragm and cutting the center to create the shape and size of the aperture.

However, one disadvantage of aperture diaphragms is that although the aperture's size and shape can be changed, the aperture cannot be adjusted from the designed size. Therefore the projected field size is not adjustable. Also, an aperture diaphragm made to fit a particular radiographic unit will not necessarily fit another radiographic unit. Because of the aperture's proximity to the radiation source (focal spot), a large area of unsharpness surrounds the radiographic image (Figure 5-4). Moving the aperture diaphragm farther away from the focal spot could theoretically solve this problem, but this is not practical. Although aperture diaphragms are still in use in some applications, their use is not as widespread as that of other types of beam-restricting devices.

CONES AND CYLINDERS

Although cones and cylinders are shaped differently (Figure 5-5), they have many of the same attributes. A **cone** or **cylinder** is essentially an aperture diaphragm that has

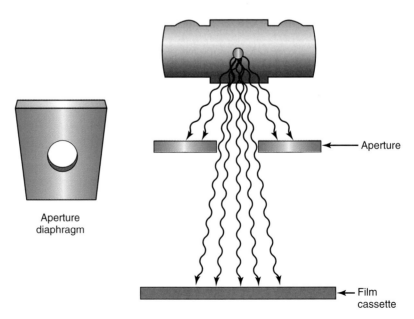

FIGURE 5-3 A commercially made aperture diaphragm.

an extended flange attached to it. The flange can vary in length and can be shaped as either a cone or a cylinder. The flange can also be made to telescope, thereby increasing its total length (Figure 5-6). Like aperture diaphragms, cones and cylinders are easy to use. They simply attach to the slots in the bottom of a collimator. Cones and cylinders limit unsharpness surrounding the radiographic image more than aperture diaphragms do, with cylinders accomplishing this task slightly better than cones (Figure 5-7). However, they are limited in terms of the sizes that are available,

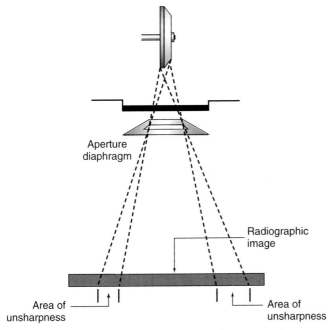

FIGURE 5-4 Radiographic image unsharpness using an aperture diaphragm.

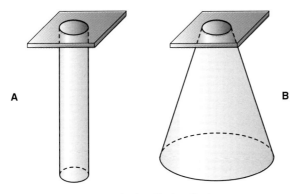

FIGURE 5-5 A, A cylinder. **B,** A cone.

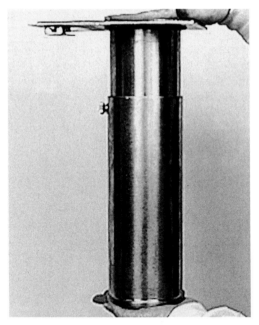

FIGURE 5-6 A telescoping cylinder. *From* Mosby's radiographic instructional series: radiographic imaging, *St Louis, 1998, Mosby.*

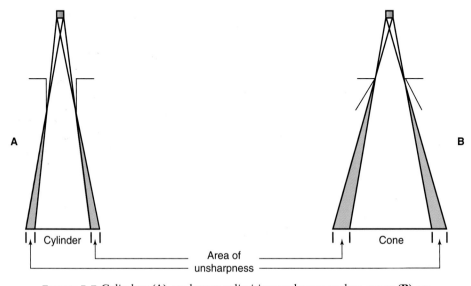

FIGURE 5-7 Cylinders (**A**) are better at limiting unsharpness than cones (**B**) are.

and they are not necessarily interchangeable among tube housings. Cones have a particular disadvantage compared with cylinders. If the angle of the flange of the cone is greater than the angle of divergence of the primary beam, the base plate or aperture diaphragm of the cone is the only metal really restricting the primary beam. Therefore cylinders generally are more popular than cones. Cones and cylinders are almost always made to produce a circular projected field, and they can be used to advantage for particular radiographic procedures (Figure 5-8).

COLLIMATORS

The most sophisticated, useful, and accepted type of beam-restricting device is the collimator. Collimators are considered the best type of beam-restricting device available for radiography. Beam restriction accomplished with the use of a collimator is referred to as *collimation.* Often, the terms *collimation* and *beam restriction* are used interchangeably.

A **collimator** has two sets of adjustable lead shutters (Figure 5-9). Each set of shutters, longitudinal and lateral, has its own control, which makes the collimator adjustable in terms of its ability to produce projected fields of varying sizes. The field shape produced by a collimator is always rectangular or square unless an aperture diaphragm, cone, or cylinder is used in conjunction with it. Collimators are equipped with a white light source and a mirror to project a light field onto the patient. This light is intended to accurately indicate where the primary beam will be projected during exposure. In case of failure of this light, an x-ray field measurement

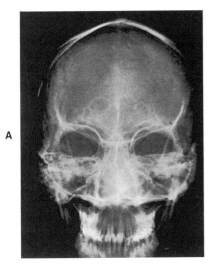
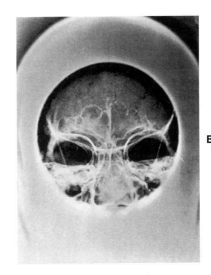

A   B

FIGURE 5-8 Radiograph of the frontal and maxillary sinuses not using a cone **(A)** and using a cone **(B).** *From* Mosby's radiographic instructional series: radiographic imaging, *St Louis, 1998, Mosby.*

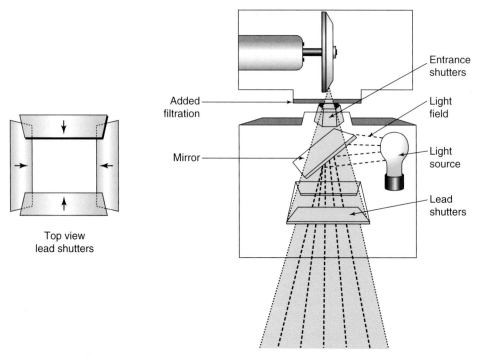

Top view
lead shutters

FIGURE 5-9 Collimators have two sets of lead shutters to change the size and shape of the primary beam.

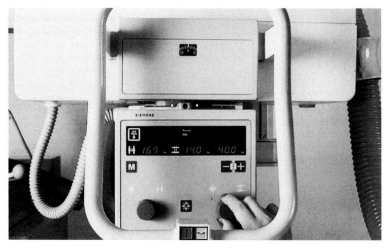

FIGURE 5-10 The x-ray field measurement guide on the front of a collimator.

guide (Figure 5-10) is present on the front of the collimator. It indicates the projected field size produced based on the adjusted size of the collimator opening at particular source-to-image receptor distances (SIDs). This helps ensure that the radiographer does not open the collimator to produce a field that is larger than the image receptor when the light is burned out. Aside from the collimator light burning out, another problem that may occur is the lack of accuracy of the light field. The mirror that reflects the light down toward the patient or the light bulb itself could be slightly out of position, projecting a light field that inaccurately indicates where the primary beam will be projected. There is a means of testing the accuracy of this light field and the location of the center of projected beam.

A plastic template with crosshairs is affixed to the bottom of the collimator to indicate where the center of the primary beam—the central ray—will be directed. This is of great assistance to the radiographer in positioning the patient accurately. Also, unsharpness around the radiographic image is best limited with a collimator.

AUTOMATIC COLLIMATORS

Automatic collimators are also called *positive beam-limiting devices,* or *PBLs.* An **automatic collimator,** or **positive beam-limiting device,** automatically limits the size and shape of the primary beam to the size and shape of the image receptor. For a number of years, automatic collimators were required by U.S. federal law (Radiation Control for Health and Safety Act of 1968, Public Law 90-602) on all new radiographic installations. A new radiographic installation was either a new piece of radiographic equipment or an old piece of radiographic equipment being installed at a site other than its original installation site. This part of Public Law 90-602 has since been rescinded, and automatic collimators are no longer a requirement on any radiographic equipment. However, they are still widely used. Automatic collimators mechanically adjust the primary beam size and shape to that of the image receptor. This adjustment decreases the likelihood that the radiographer will increase the size of the primary beam to a field larger than the image receptor, thereby increasing the patient's radiation exposure. PBL devices were seen as a way of protecting patients from overexposure to radiation. However, it should be noted that automatic collimators have an override mechanism that allows the radiographer to disengage the PBL feature.

Practical Tip

Limiting Field Size to Image Receptor Size

The size of the projected radiation field should never exceed the size of the image receptor. This will ensure patient protection from excessive radiation exposure while also improving image quality.

Radiographic Grids

The radiographic grid was invented in 1913 by Gustave Bucky. A **grid** is a device that has interspaced lead lines intended to absorb scatter radiation emitted from the patient before it strikes the image receptor, thereby increasing radiographic contrast. Grids are placed between the patient and the image receptor. Grids are valuable in the practice of radiography and have undergone many physical changes since their inception. They work well to improve radiographic contrast, but they are not perfect devices.

As scatter radiation leaves the patient, a significant amount of it is directed at the image receptor. As stated previously, scatter radiation exposure is detrimental to radiographic quality because it adds unwanted density to the radiograph without adding any patient information. Scatter radiation decreases radiographic contrast. Ideally, grids would absorb all scattered photons directed toward the image receptor and would allow all transmitted photons emitted from the patient to pass from the patient to the image receptor. Unfortunately, this does not happen (Figure 5-11). However, when used properly, grids can greatly increase the contrast of the radiographic image.

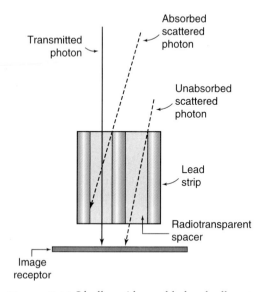

FIGURE 5-11 Ideally, grids would absorb all scattered radiation and allow all transmitted photons to reach the film. In reality, however, some scattered photons are allowed to pass through to the film, and some transmitted photons are absorbed.

Scatter Radiation and Image Quality

Scatter radiation adds unwanted density to the radiograph and decreases image quality.

Grid Construction

Grids contain thin lead lines that have a precise height, thickness, and space between them. Radiolucent **interspace material** separates the lead lines. Interspace material typically is made of aluminum. The lead lines and interspace material of the grid are covered by an aluminum front and back panel.

Grid construction can be described by its grid frequency. **Grid frequency** expresses the number of lead lines per unit length, usually either in inches, centimeters, or both. Grid frequencies can range in value from 25 to 45 lines/cm (60 to 110 lines/inch). A typical value for grid frequency, for example, might be 40 lines/cm or 103 lines/inch. Another way of describing grid construction is by its grid ratio. **Grid ratio** is defined as the ratio of the height of the lead lines to the distance between them (Figure 5-12). Grid ratio can also be expressed mathematically as follows:

$$\text{Grid ratio} = h/D$$

where *h* is the height of the lead lines and *D* is the distance between them.

Grid ratios range from 4:1 to 16:1. High-ratio grids remove more scatter radiation than lower-ratio grids and thus increase radiographic contrast.

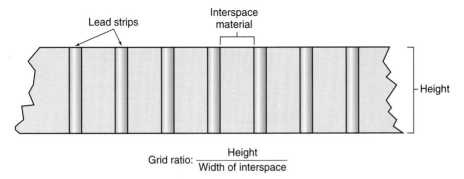

FIGURE 5-12 Grid ratio is the ratio of the height of the lead lines to the distance between them.

Important Relationship

Grid Ratio and Radiographic Contrast

As grid ratio increases, radiographic contrast increases; as grid ratio decreases, radiographic contrast decreases.

Information about a grid's construction is contained on a label placed on the tube side of the grid. This label usually states the type of interspace material used, grid frequency, grid ratio, grid size, and information about the range of SIDs that can be used with the grid. This is important information that the radiographer should read before using the grid because these factors influence grid performance.

GRID PATTERN

Grid pattern refers to the linear pattern of the lead lines of a grid. Two types of grid pattern exist: linear and crossed or cross-hatched. A **linear grid** has lead lines that run in only one direction (Figure 5-13). Linear grids are the most popular in terms of grid pattern because they allow angulation of the x-ray tube along the

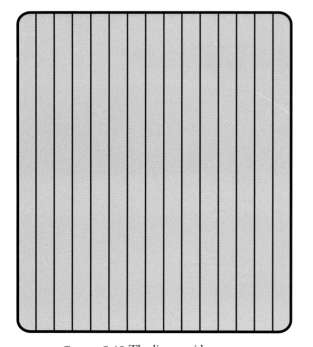

FIGURE 5-13 The linear grid pattern.

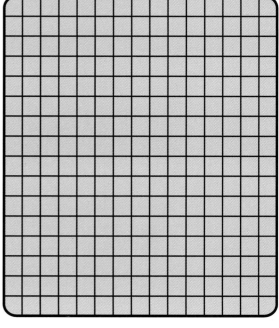

FIGURE 5-14 The crossed or cross-hatched grid pattern.

length of the lead lines. A **crossed** or **cross-hatched grid** has lead lines that run at a right angle to one another (Figure 5-14). Crossed grids remove more scattered photons than linear grids because they contain more lead strips, oriented in two directions. However, applications are limited with a crossed grid because the x-ray tube cannot be angled against the grid without producing grid cutoff. Grid cutoff is undesirable and is discussed later in this chapter.

GRID FOCUS

Grid focus refers to the orientation of the lead lines to one another. Two types of grid focus exist: parallel (nonfocused) and focused. A **parallel** or **nonfocused grid** has lead lines that run parallel to one another (Figure 5-15). Parallel grids are used primarily in fluoroscopy. A **focused grid** has lead lines that are angled to approximately match the angle of divergence of the primary beam. The advantage of focused grids compared with parallel grids is that focused grids allow more transmitted photons to reach the image receptor. When the angle of divergence of the primary beam is simulated (Figure 5-16), transmitted photons are more likely to pass through a focused grid to reach the film than they are to pass through a parallel grid (Figure 5-17).

Important Relationship

Focused versus Parallel Grids

Focused grids have lead lines that are angled to approximately match the divergence of the primary beam. Thus focused grids allow more transmitted photons to reach the image receptor than parallel grids.

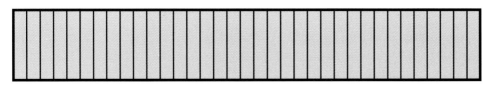

FIGURE 5-15 The parallel, or nonfocused, type of grid focus.

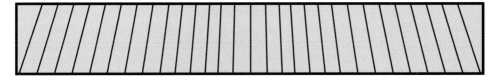

FIGURE 5-16 The focused type of grid focus.

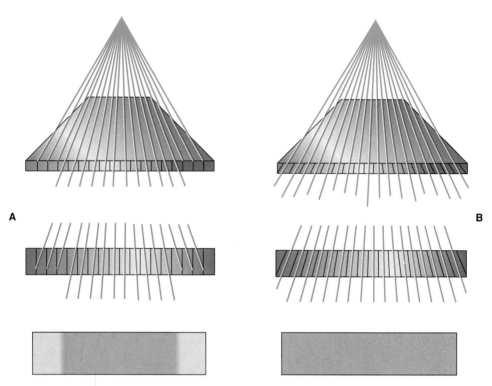

FIGURE 5-17 Comparison of transmitted photons passing through a parallel grid **(A)** and a focused grid **(B).**

If imaginary lines were drawn from each of the lead lines in a linear focused grid, these lines would come together to form an imaginary line. This imaginary line is called the **convergent line** (Figure 5-18). If imaginary lines were drawn from each of the lead lines in a crossed focused grid, these lines would come together to form an imaginary point. This imaginary point is called the **convergent point** (Figure 5-19). Both the convergent line and convergent point are important because they determine the focal distance of a focused grid. The **focal distance** is the distance between the grid and the convergent line or convergent point. The focal distance is important because it is used to determine the focal range of a focused grid. The **focal range** is the recommended range of SIDs that can be used with a focused grid. The convergent line or point always falls within the focal range (Figure 5-20). For example, a common focal range is 36 to 42 inches, with a focal distance of 40 inches. Another common focal range is 66 to 74 inches, with a focal distance of 72 inches. Using the grid outside of this range of SIDs causes grid cutoff. Because the lead lines in a parallel grid are not angled, they have a focal range extending from a minimum SID to infinity.

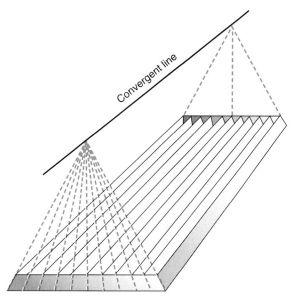

FIGURE 5-18 Imaginary lines drawn above a linear focused grid from each lead line meet to form a convergent line.

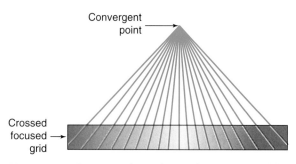

FIGURE 5-19 Imaginary lines drawn above a crossed focused grid from each lead line meet to form a convergent point.

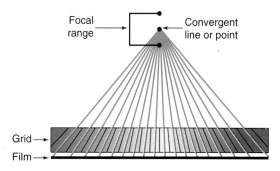

FIGURE 5-20 The convergent line or point of a focused grid falls within a focal range.

Important Relationship

Grid Focal Distance and Grid Cutoff

To eliminate the production of grid cutoff, the radiographer should use an SID within the focal range labeled on the grid.

Practical Tip

Grid Selection

Grids differ from one another in performance, especially regarding grid ratio and focal distance. Before using a grid, the radiographer must determine the grid ratio so that the appropriate exposure factors can be selected. Also, the radiographer must be aware of the focal range of focused grids, or the minimum SID of parallel grids, so that the appropriate SID is selected. In addition, if the grid is mounted to a cassette, the film-screen speed should be determined before the exposure factors are selected. Box 5-1 lists attributes of the typical grid used in radiography.

BOX 5-1 *The Typical Grid*

Is linear instead of crossed
Is focused instead of parallel
Is of midratio (6:1 to 12:1)
Has a focal range that includes an SID of 40 inches

Types of Grids

Grids are available for use by the radiographer in several forms, and they match the available sizes of image receptors. A **wafer grid** is used by simply placing it on top of an imaging receptor. Wafer grids typically are taped to the imaging receptor to prevent them from sliding off of the cassette during the radiographic procedure. A **grid cassette** is an imaging receptor that has a grid permanently mounted to its front surface. Grid cassettes are versatile for this reason, but the film inside must be taken out and the cassette reloaded before the grid can be used again. A **grid cap** contains a permanently mounted grid and allows the imaging receptor to slide behind it. This is useful because the grid is secure and many imaging receptors can be interchanged behind the grid before processing the film. One company markets an innovative form of grid for use with portable radiographic examinations. It has a grid on one side over a pocket that the cassette slides into. It is intended to make grid use easier for the radiographer and more comfortable for the patient.

Radiographic grids are also located inside radiographic tables and wall units. Inside radiographic tables, these grids are made to move during exposure. These grids usually have dimensions of 17 × 17 inches so that a 14 × 17 inch cassette can be positioned under the grid either lengthwise or crosswise, depending on the examination requirements. Inside wall units, grids may be either moving or stationary.

These grids typically measure either 14×17 inches or 17×17 inches. A circular grid is also used in fluoroscopic equipment as part of the fluoroscopic tower.

Grid Performance

The purpose of using grids in radiography is to increase radiographic contrast. Thus the best measure of how well a grid performs is the contrast improvement factor. The **contrast improvement factor** is expressed mathematically as follows:

$$K = \frac{\text{Radiographic contrast with a grid}}{\text{Radiographic contrast without a grid}}$$

where K signifies the contrast improvement factor. This is a fundamental formula in terms of quality assurance applications.

A much more practical aspect of grid performance is the Bucky factor, or grid conversion factor (GCF). Named for the inventor of grids, the **Bucky factor** can be used to indicate the changes in exposure factors that must be made when changing from not using a grid to using a grid, or vice versa, or when changing the grid ratio. Changing exposure factors based on grid use and grid ratio is important because grids have a profound effect on radiographic density.

Important Relationship

Grid Ratio and Radiographic Density

As grid ratio increases, radiographic density decreases; as grid ratio decreases, radiographic density increases.

Table 5-2 presents specific grid ratios and recommended changes in mAs.

TABLE 5-2   THE BUCKY FACTOR/GRID CONVERSION FACTOR (GCF)

Grid Ratio	mAs Increase	Bucky Factor/GCF
5:1	$2\times$	2
6:1	$3\times$	3
8:1	$4\times$	4
12:1	$5\times$	5
16:1	$6\times$	6

When a grid is added to the imaging receptor, mAs must be increased by the factors indicated to maintain radiographic density. This requires multiplication by the Bucky factor/GCF for a particular grid ratio.

 X *Mathematical Application*

Using a Grid

If a radiographer produced a knee radiograph with a nongrid exposure using 10 mAs and on the next exposure wanted to use an 8:1 grid, what mAs should be used to produce a radiograph of the same density?

Nongrid exposure = 10 mAs
8:1 grid
GCF = 4 (from Table 5-2)

$$GCF = \frac{mAs \text{ with a grid}}{mAs \text{ without the grid}}$$

Step One: $4 = \dfrac{mAs}{10}$

Step Two: $(4)(10) = mAs$

Step Three: $40 = mAs$ with a grid

NOTE: mAs must be increased by a factor of 4 to 40 mAs.

Likewise, if a radiographer chooses to not use a grid in a situation in which one typically is used, he or she must decrease mAs by the factor indicated to maintain radiographic density. This requires division by the Bucky factor/GCF for a particular grid ratio.

 X *Mathematical Application*

Not Using a Grid

If a radiographer produced a knee radiograph using a 16:1 grid and 60 mAs and on the next exposure wanted to use a nongrid exposure, what mAs should be used to produce a radiograph of the same density?

Grid exposure = 60 mAs
16:1 grid
GCF = 6 (from Table 5-2)

$$GCF = \frac{mAs \text{ with a grid}}{mAs \text{ without the grid}}$$

Step One: $6 = \dfrac{60}{\text{mAs}}$

Step Two: $(\text{mAs})(6) = \left(\dfrac{60}{\text{mAs}} \right)(\text{mAs})$

Step Three: $\text{mAs} = (60)\left(\dfrac{1}{6} \right)$

Step Four: $\text{mAs} = 10$

NOTE: mAs must be decreased by a factor of 6 to 10 mAs.

The Bucky factor is also useful when changing grid ratios. The Bucky factor for the new grid is divided by the Bucky factor for the original grid, and this result is then multiplied by the mAs that was used for the original grid.

X Mathematical Application

Increasing the Grid Ratio

If a radiographer performed a routine portable kidney, ureter, and bladder (KUB) examination using 30 mAs with a 6:1 grid, what mAs should be used if a 12:1 grid were used?

30 mAs, 6:1 grid, Bucky factor = 3
_____ mAs, 12:1 grid, Bucky factor = 5

$$\dfrac{\textbf{mAs}_1}{\textbf{mAs}_2} = \dfrac{\textbf{BF}_1}{\textbf{BF}_2}$$

Step One: $\dfrac{30}{\text{mAs}_2} = \dfrac{3}{5}$

Step Two: Simply cross multiply:
$(\text{mAs}_2)(3) = (30)(5)$

Step Three: $\text{mAs}_2 = \dfrac{(30)(5)}{3}$

Step Four: $\text{mAs}_2 = 50 \text{ mAs}$

An example demonstrating the result of decreasing grid ratio follows.

X *Mathematical Application*

Decreasing the Grid Ratio

If a radiographer used 37.5 mAs with an 8:1 grid, what mAs should be used with a 5:1 grid?

37.5 mAs, 8:1 grid, Bucky factor = 4
_____ mAs, 5:1 grid, Bucky factor = 2

$$\frac{mAs_1}{mAs_2} = \frac{BF_1}{BF_2}$$

Step One: $\dfrac{37.5}{mAs_2} = \dfrac{4}{2}$

Step Two: $(mAs_2)(4) = (37.5)(2)$

Step Three: $mAs_2 = \dfrac{(37.5)(2)}{4}$

Step Four: $mAs_2 = 18.75$ mAs

It is important to note that patient dose is increased because of the following:

1. Using a grid compared with not using a grid
2. Using a higher ratio grid

This increase in patient dose is caused by the increase in mAs required to maintain density on the radiograph. This increase in patient dose is significant, as the numbers for the Bucky factor indicate.

Important Relationship

Grid Ratio and Patient Dose

As grid ratio increases, patient dose increases; as grid ratio decreases, patient dose decreases.

Grid Cutoff

In addition to the disadvantage of increased patient dose associated with grid use, another disadvantage is the possibility of grid cutoff. **Grid cutoff** is defined as a decrease in the number of transmitted photons that reach the film because of some misalignment of the grid. The primary radiographic effect of grid cutoff is a decrease in radiographic density. Grid cutoff generally requires that the radiographer repeat the radiograph, thereby increasing patient dose yet again. The likelihood of grid cutoff depends on the ratio of the grid being used.

Important Relationship

Grid Ratio and Grid Cutoff

As grid ratio increases, the likelihood of grid cutoff increases; as grid ratio decreases, the likelihood of grid cutoff decreases.

TYPES OF GRID CUTOFF

Three types of grid cutoff can occur as a result of errors in grid use. To eliminate grid cutoff, the radiographer must have a thorough understanding of the importance of proper grid placement in relation to the image receptor and x-ray tube.

Upside Down Focused

Upside down focused grid cutoff occurs when a focused grid is placed upside down on the image receptor so that the tube side of the grid is facing the image receptor and not the x-ray tube. This appears radiographically as a plus density (dark) strip down the center of the radiograph (Figure 5-21). Photons easily pass through the center of the grid because the lead lines are perpendicular to the image receptor surface. Lead lines that are more peripheral to the center are angled more to match the divergent angle of the primary beam and thus absorb the photons readily.

Important Relationship

Upside Down Focused Grids and Grid Cutoff

Placing a focused grid upside down on the image receptor causes a plus density (dark) strip to appear down the center of the radiograph.

Lateral Decentering

Lateral decentering grid cutoff is the most common type of cutoff and can occur in more than one way. For example, exposing the grid against its lead lines occurs either by angling the tube against the lead lines or by the grid itself being angled during exposure (Figure 5-22). The latter is referred to as an *off-level grid*. Another way in which lateral decentering can occur is by not placing the central ray to the

FIGURE 5-21 A radiograph produced with an upside down focused grid.

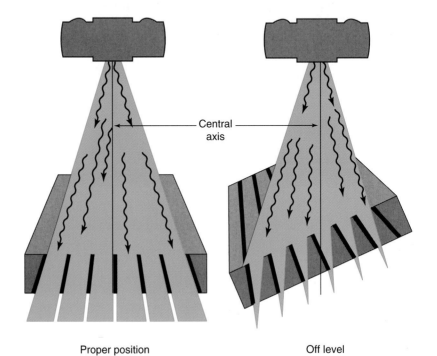

FIGURE 5-22 An off-level grid can cause lateral decentering grid cutoff.

center of a focused grid. Because of the arrangement of the lead lines of the focused grid, the divergence of the primary beam does not match the angle of these lead strips when not centered to the focused grid (Figure 5-23). This is referred to as an *off-center grid.* Lateral decentering appears radiographically as an overall loss of density (Figure 5-24).

Important Relationship

Lateral Decentering and Grid Cutoff

Angling the x-ray tube across the grid lines or angling the grid itself during exposure produces an overall decrease in density on the radiograph.

Distance Decentering

Distance decentering occurs when using a focused grid outside of the recommended focal range (SID) or when using a parallel grid at less than the recommended minimum SID. Focused grid distance decentering can occur as either far-distance

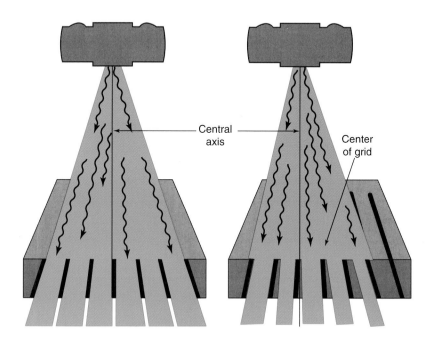

Proper position   Off center

FIGURE 5-23 Centering lateral to the center of a focused grid can cause lateral decentering grid cutoff.

FIGURE 5-24 Radiograph demonstrating lateral decentering grid cutoff.

decentering or near-distance decentering. Far-distance decentering occurs when an SID that is greater than the recommended focal range of the grid is used. Near-distance decentering occurs when an SID that is less than the recommended focal range of the grid is used. Both far- and near-distance decentering and parallel grid distance decentering appear the same radiographically—as a loss of density at the periphery of the film (Figure 5-25).

Important Relationship

Distance Decentering and Grid Cutoff

Using an SID outside of the focal range creates a loss of density at the periphery of the radiograph.

Grid cutoff often is produced by more than one problem at a time. Lateral decentering can combine with distance decentering to cause grid cutoff. This produces a radiograph that has a plus (dark) density on one side and a minus density (light) on the other (Figure 5-26). Lateral and distance decentering often occur during portable radiographic examinations. The radiographer should pay close attention to the placement of the radiographic grid during these types of procedures.

FIGURE 5-25 Radiograph demonstrating distance decentering grid cutoff.

FIGURE 5-26 Radiograph demonstrating combined lateral and distance decentering grid cutoff.

Moving Grids

A mechanism to make grids move during radiographic exposure was invented in 1920 by Hollis Potter. Today, such a system generally is called a **Bucky**, but its true name is a Potter-Bucky diaphragm, combining the surnames of Potter and the inventor of the grid. The advantage of a moving grid compared with a stationary grid is the elimination of grid lines from the radiographic image. Buckys are found in radiographic tables and in upright wall units, although some wall units still use only stationary grids.

RECIPROCATING GRIDS

The reciprocating motion is the most common type of grid used today. Grid motion is controlled electrically by the x-ray exposure switch. The grid moves back and forth in a lateral direction over the image receptor during the entire exposure. This type of motion is somewhat limited by very fast exposure times because the grid must change direction. This problem has been solved with the use of a high-speed Bucky. A **high-speed Bucky** is a reciprocating grid that is capable of moving fast enough to eliminate grid lines from being imaged, even with exposure times as short as 0.0083 second.

DISADVANTAGES

Moving grids present some disadvantages compared with stationary grids. Despite these disadvantages, moving grids are more widely used than stationary grids. One disadvantage is that moving grid technology is more expensive than stationary grid technology. This may be why some radiographic wall units still use only stationary grids. Moving grids also vibrate the radiographic tabletop to a small degree during exposure. This vibration can be a little disconcerting to patients, but it is not noticeable with most units. The mechanism that causes the grid to move is sometimes prone to failure. This propensity is a minor consideration because if a moving grid does not move, it is a stationary grid and is still sufficient for most examinations. Using a moving grid causes a small degree of lateral decentering grid cutoff because the grid is moving laterally compared with the stationary primary beam. This may cause the radiographer to use slightly more mAs than would be used with a stationary grid, thereby increasing patient dose slightly. However, this is considered inconsequential to patient exposure. Bucky mechanisms cause an increase in object-to-image receptor distance (OID), which increases magnification and decreases recorded detail. The thickness of Bucky mechanisms generally ranges from about 2.5 to 4.0 inches. However, the benefit of eliminating grid lines out weighs the minimal increase in magnification and decrease in recorded detail.

Grid Use

Using a grid has the disadvantage of requiring an increase in mAs, consequently increasing patient dose. However, using a grid has the advantage of increasing radiographic contrast. These are two competing entities: patient dose and radiographic quality. The radiographer's task is to produce a high-quality radiograph while delivering the smallest radiation dose to the patient. Some guidance on this issue as it pertains to grids is available. In general, a grid is used when the anatomic part size exceeds 9 cm in thickness. In other words, the production of scatter radiation in a part exceeding 9 cm is considered great enough to significantly decrease radiographic contrast to the point that using a grid outweighs the increase in patient dose that the grid will require. This is still a judgment that should be left to the discretion of the individual radiographer or departmental standards.

A good example of the dilemma of grid use as it impacts patient dose and radiographic quality is the adult knee. The thickness of the adult knee from its anterior surface to its posterior surface is usually about 10 cm. However, knee radiographs can be produced using a variety of imaging techniques. Knee radiographs are produced with and without grids, with fast screens and with detail screens, and with every combination of each that is possible. Clearly, the tradeoff between contrast improvement and patient dose is one that radiographers handle in different ways. Fortunately, there is an obvious benefit in the guidance of using grids in parts exceeding 9 cm in thickness, as evidenced by the other kinds of examinations for which grids are used. In general, the greater the part thickness, the more benefit there is in using a grid.

Also, several sources provide some guidance in terms of what grid ratios should be used according to the kVp value used (Table 5-3). Such a system states that increasing kVp produces lower contrast, so high values of kVp require higher grid ratios.

The Air Gap Technique

The **air gap technique** is used instead of a grid but for the same purpose that grids are used, and it requires that the patient be positioned some distance away from the film. It has been recommended that a 5-inch air gap will improve radiographic contrast about the same as a 7:1 grid for thin patients and that a 10-inch air gap will improve radiographic contrast about the same as a 15:1 grid for thin patients, but not as well as with thick patients.[1] The classic example of how this occurs in normal radiographic positioning is with the lateral position of the cervical spine in adults (Figure 5-27). Because the shoulder in this position is against the image receptor,

TABLE 5-3 **RECOMMENDED GRID RATIOS BASED ON kVp USED**

kVp	Grid Ratio
Below 90	8:1 or below
90-125	12:1
125 and above	16:1

[1]Curry TS, Dowdy JE, Murry RC: *Christensen's physics of diagnostic radiology*, ed 4, Philadelphia, 1990, Lea & Febiger.

a natural air gap between the image receptor and neck exists. The adult neck as measured in this aspect typically exceeds 9 cm, requiring the use of a grid. However, a grid is not necessary because of the air gap between the image receptor and part.

There are two reasons why it is believed the air gap technique works in place of a grid. By increasing the OID, scattered photons simply miss the film because of the angle they are traveling at in relation to the grid lines. These scattered photons would otherwise decrease radiographic contrast if they did indeed strike the image receptor. Also, it is believed that the air between the part and the film has some minimal effect in filtering scattered photons before they strike the film.

Two advantages of the air gap technique are that grid lines are not imaged on the radiograph (although this would be negated by use of a moving grid) and the patient receives a smaller dose than he or she would with the use of a grid. An obvious disadvantage is the increase in OID that the technique requires. This increase in OID increases magnification and decreases recorded detail.

Practical Tip

OID and the Air Gap Technique

Using an increased OID is a necessity for the air gap technique. However, this decreases image quality. To decrease magnification and increase recorded detail when using the air gap technique, the radiographer must increase SID.

The air gap technique has been used successfully in chest radiography by using SIDs as great as 120 inches (10 ft). It can also be used successfully in some instances when a radiographer needs a grid but does not have one and cannot immediately obtain one. Such instances sometimes arise in emergency and trauma situations.

Table 5-4 summarizes important relationships regarding the use of radiographic grids.

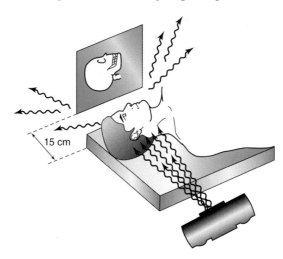

FIGURE 5-27 The air gap technique used in radiography of the lateral cervical spine.

TABLE 5-4   RADIOGRAPHIC GRIDS

Increased Factor	Result
Grid ratio*	Contrast **increases.**
	Patient dose **increases.**
	The likelihood of grid cutoff **increases.**

*mAs adjusted to maintain density.

 FILM CRITIQUE

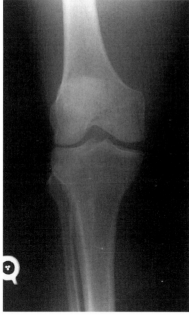

FIGURE 5-28 Image A was produced using 70 kVp, 100 mA at 0.016 s, 400 speed film-screen combination, a 40-inch source-to-image receptor distance, and no grid.

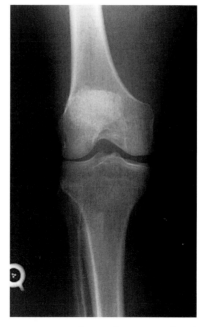

FIGURE 5-29 Image B was produced using 70 kVp, 50 mA at 0.160 s, 400 speed film-screen combination, a 40-inch source-to-image receptor distance, and a 12:1 grid ratio.

1. Evaluate each radiograph and discuss its quality.

2. For each image, evaluate its exposure variables and discuss their effect on the quality of the image, regardless of whether it is apparent on the radiograph.

3. For each image, identify any adjustments that could be made in the exposure factors to produce an optimal image.

Review Questions

1. The projected shape of the unrestricted primary beam is
   A. square.
   B. rectangular.
   C. circular.
   D. elliptical.

2. The purpose of beam restricting devices is to _____ by changing the size and shape of the primary beam.
   A. decrease patient dose
   B. decrease scatter radiation
   C. decrease the density
   D. increase the contrast

3. The best type of beam-restricting device is the
   A. cone.
   B. aperture diaphragm.
   C. cylinder.
   D. collimator.

4. Of the beam-restricting devices listed in question 3, which two are most similar to one another?
   A. A and B
   B. A and C
   C. B and C
   D. B and D

5. The purpose of automatic collimation is to ensure that
   A. the intensity of scatter production is minimized.
   B. the field size does not exceed the image receptor size.
   C. maximal recorded detail and contrast are achieved.
   D. radiographic density is maintained.

6. When collimating significantly
   A. mAs should be increased.
   B. kVp should be increased.
   C. mAs should be decreased.
   D. kVp should be decreased.

7. Which one of the following will increase as collimation increases?
   A. Density
   B. Scatter production
   C. Fog
   D. Contrast

8. Which of the following is true of positive beam-limiting devices?
   A. They are required on all radiographic installations.
   B. They are required on all new radiographic installations.
   C. They have never been required on radiographic installations.
   D. They were once required on new radiographic installations.

9. The purpose of a grid in radiography is to
   A. increase density.
   B. increase contrast.
   C. decrease patient dose.
   D. increase recorded detail.

10. Grid ratio is defined as the ratio of the
    A. height of the lead lines to the distance between them.
    B. width of the lead lines to their height.
    C. number of lead lines to their width.
    D. width of the lead lines to the width of the interspace material.

11. Compared with parallel grids, focused grids
    A. have a greater grid frequency and lead content.
    B. produce greater scatter absorption and contrast.
    C. have a wider range of grid ratios and frequencies.
    D. allow more transmitted photons to pass to the film.

12. With which one of the following grids would a convergent line be formed if imaginary lines from its grid lines were drawn in space above it?
    A. Linear focused
    B. Crossed focused
    C. Linear parallel
    D. Crossed parallel

13. If 15 mAs were used to produce a particular level of radiographic density without a grid, what mAs would be needed to produce that same level of density using a 16:1 grid?
    A. 45
    B. 60
    C. 90
    D. 105

14. Grid cutoff, regardless of the type, is most recognizable radiographically because of inadequate
    A. contrast.
    B. recorded detail.
    C. density.
    D. positioning.

15. Distance decentering grid cutoff occurs by using an SID that is not
    A. within the focal range of the grid.
    B. equal to the focal distance of the grid.

C. at the level of the convergent line of the grid.
D. at the level of the convergent point of the grid.

16. The type of motion most used for moving grids today is
    A. longitudinal.
    B. reciprocating.
    C. circular.
    D. single stroke.

17. A grid should be used whenever the anatomic part size exceeds
    A. 3 cm
    B. 6 cm
    C. 9 cm
    D. 12 cm

18. The air gap technique requires an increase in _____ compared with using a grid.
    A. kVp
    B. mAs
    C. SID
    D. OID

CHAPTER 6

Image Receptors

RADIOGRAPHIC FILM

Film Construction
Latent Image Formation
Types of Film
    Direct-Exposure Film
    Screen Film
Film Characteristics
    Film Speed, Film Contrast, and Exposure Latitude
    Spectral Sensitivity
    Crossover

INTENSIFYING SCREENS

Purpose and Function
Luminescence
Screen Construction
Screen Characteristics
    Types of Phosphors
    Screen Speed
    Screen Speed and Recorded Detail
Screen Maintenance

CASSETTES

FILM CRITIQUE

REVIEW QUESTIONS

OBJECTIVES

1 Define all of the key terms in this chapter.

2 State all of the important relationships in this chapter.

3 Describe the layers that make up radiographic film.

4 Explain how the latent image is formed.

5 Differentiate between direct-exposure film and screen film, single and double emulsion.

6 Describe film characteristics, including speed, contrast, latitude, spectral sensitivity, and crossover.

7 Describe the purpose and function of intensifying screens.

8 Describe the layers that make up intensifying screens.

9 Explain how screens can be characterized based on the type of phosphor, spectral emission, and screen speed.

10 Demonstrate use of the intensification factor (IF).

11 Demonstrate use of the mAs conversion formula for screens.

12 Describe factors that affect screen speed.

13 Explain the effect screen speed has on recorded detail.

14 Describe two major intensifying screen maintenance concerns.

15 Describe the function and construction of a cassette.

KEY TERMS

supercoat
emulsion
silver halide
base layer
latent image
manifest image
latent image centers
direct-exposure film
screen film
double-emulsion film
single-emulsion screen film
speed
spectral sensitivity
spectral emission
spectral matching
crossover
intensifying screen

phosphor
luminescence
fluorescence
phosphorescence
protective layer
phosphor layer
reflecting layer
absorbing layer
base
rare earth elements
screen speed
intensification factor (IF)
relative speed
mAs conversion formula for screens
quantum mottle
film-screen contact

Double-emulsion radiographic film, as used in a cassette with intensifying screens, is the most common image receptor used in radiography today. The intensifying screens absorb the transmitted x-rays and produce light, which exposes the film. The film records the image based on the pattern of transmitted x-rays and the light produced by the intensifying screens. The cassette is the rigid, light-tight container that holds the screens and film in close contact.

Radiographic Film

Several types of radiographic film are used in today's medical imaging department, depending on the specific application. Film manufacturers produce film in a variety of sizes, ranging from 20 × 25 cm (8 × 10 inches) to 35 × 43 cm (14 × 17 inches) (Figure 6-1).

FILM CONSTRUCTION

The composition of film can be described in layers (Figure 6-2). The outside layer is called the *supercoat*. The **supercoat** is a durable protective layer that is intended to prevent damage to the sensitive emulsion layer underneath it.

The next layer down is the emulsion layer. The **emulsion** layer is the radiation- and light-sensitive layer of the film. The emulsion of film consists of silver halide crystals suspended in gelatin. **Silver halide** is the material that is sensitive to radiation and light. Although the precise formulations of silver halide used by radiographic film manufacturers are held as proprietary information, it generally is believed that silver bromide (AgBr) and silver iodide (AgI) make up the emulsion layer of film. In addition, it is generally believed that silver bromide constitutes 90% to 99% of the silver halide in film emulsions and that silver iodide makes up the remaining 1% to 10%.

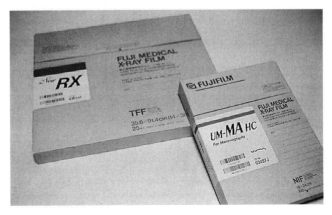

FIGURE 6-1 Radiographic film is available in a variety of types and sizes.

A fairly recent innovation that has been incorporated into manufacturing film is what has become known as *tabular grain* (or *T-grain*) technology. Instead of using randomly shaped silver halide crystals in the emulsion layers, T-grain film uses flat silver halide crystals that can be dispersed more evenly in the emulsion layer gelatin than conventional crystals (Figure 6-3). This is intended to increase the recorded detail of the radiographs produced with this film. This technology has been well accepted by the radiography industry, and T-grain film is widely used today.

The final layer of film is the base layer. The **base layer** is polyester (plastic) that gives the film physical stability. The emulsion layer is fairly fragile and needs this plastic base so that the film can be handled and processed, yet remain physically strong after processing. Most film used in radiographic procedures has a blue dye or tint added to the base layer to decrease eye strain in persons viewing the finished radiograph.

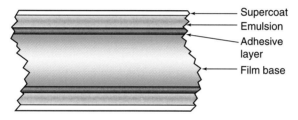

Supercoat
Emulsion
Adhesive layer
Film base

FIGURE 6-2 Composition of radiographic film.

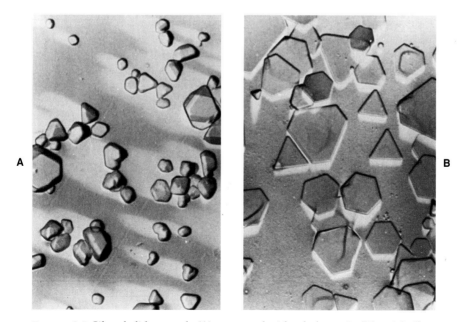

A

B

FIGURE 6-3 Silver halide crystals **(A)** compared with tabular grain (T-grain) silver halide crystals **(B).** *Courtesy Eastman Kodak.*

Between the emulsion layer and the base layer is an adhesive. The adhesive simply adheres one layer of the film to another.

LATENT IMAGE FORMATION

The term **latent image** refers to that image which exists on film after that film has been exposed but before it has been processed. Radiographic processing changes the latent image into a manifest image. The term **manifest image** refers to the image that exists on film after exposure and processing. The manifest image typically is called the *radiographic image.*

The specific way in which the latent image is formed is not really known, but the Gurney-Mott theory of latent image formation is most widely believed to be the manner in which this process happens. To explain latent image formation, it is necessary to describe what happens at the molecular level in the emulsion layer of film. Specifically, it is necessary to describe what happens to silver halide crystals when exposure to x-rays and light occurs. Silver halide is made up of both silver bromide and silver iodide. However, because silver bromide (AgBr) is the primary constituent of the silver halide in the emulsion layer of film, discussion here is of silver bromide only. The process by which the latent image is formed is precisely the same for silver iodide as it is for silver bromide.

Latent image formation as described here is depicted in Figure 6-4. Silver (Ag) and bromide (Br) are bound together as a molecule in such a way that they share an electron. This electron is shared through ionic bonding because silver is a transitional atom, having only one atom in its outer shell, and it tends to either lose it or share it. The silver in AgBr is in effect an ion because it shares only its outer-shell electron with bromide. Energy in the form of x-rays or light is absorbed by the emulsion layer(s) of radiographic film. This energy absorption raises the conductivity level of the electrons in the AgBr molecules, and these electrons move faster as a result. If enough energy is absorbed by a particular AgBr molecule, the bromide will lose an electron. The silver, in effect, becomes a positive ion because it loses its shared electron to the newly ionized bromide.

Physical imperfections in the lattice or architecture of the emulsion layers occur during the film manufacturing process. These imperfections are called *sensitivity specks.* Each sensitivity speck serves as an electron trap, trapping the electrons lost by the bromide when x-ray or light exposure occurs. Therefore these sensitivity specks become negatively charged.

Because the sensitivity specks are negatively charged, the positive silver ions that have been liberated from bromide are attracted to them. Every silver ion that gets attracted to an electron becomes neutralized by that electron, therefore becoming metallic silver. The more x-ray or light exposure in a particular area of the film, the more electrons and silver available to be attracted to the sensitivity specks. The bromide that has been liberated by x-ray or light exposure is neutral and is simply absorbed into the emulsion.

Several sensitivity specks with many silver ions attracted to them become **latent image centers.** These latent image centers appear as radiographic density on the

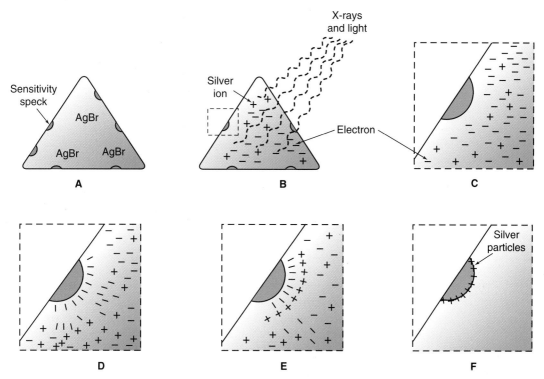

FIGURE 6-4 Latent image formation theory. **A,** Before exposure, silver halide (AgBr and AgI) is suspended in gelatin in the emulsion layer. Sensitivity specks exist as physical imperfections in the film lattice. **B,** Exposure to x-rays and light ionizes the silver halide. **C,** Negatively charged electrons and positively charged silver ions float freely in the emulsion gelatin. **D,** Sensitivity specks trap electrons. **E,** Each trapped electron attracts a silver ion. **F,** Silver clumps around the sensitivity specks.

manifest image after processing. It is believed that for a latent image center to appear, it must contain at least three sensitivity specks containing at least three silver atoms each. The more exposure to the film, the more metallic silver seen on the radiograph as radiographic density.

Important Relationship

Sensitivity Specks and Latent Image Centers

Sensitivity specks serve as the focal point for the development of latent image centers. After exposure, these specks trap the free electrons and then attract and neutralize the positive silver ions. After enough silver is neutralized, the specks become a latent image center and are converted to black metallic silver after processing.

TYPES OF FILM

Two general types of film are used in diagnostic imaging: direct-exposure film and screen film. Direct-exposure film is used without intensifying screens, whereas screen film, used with intensifying screens, is available in single- or double-emulsion varieties.

Direct-Exposure Film

Direct-exposure film is often called *nonscreen film*. It is intended to be used in a cardboard holder (instead of a cassette) and without intensifying screens. It has a single emulsion that is significantly thicker than screen film and requires more development time. Compared with screen film, direct-exposure film requires notably more exposure and may need to be manually processed. Although still commonly used for intraoral dental radiography, direct-exposure medical film and direct-exposure radiography generally are considered technologies of the past.

Screen Film

Screen film is the most widely used radiographic film today. As its name implies, it is intended to be used with one or two intensifying screens. Compared with direct-exposure film, screen film is more sensitive to light and less sensitive to x-rays. The emulsion layers are thinner than those of direct-exposure film and require less development time. Screen film requires less x-ray exposure and can be either manually or automatically processed. Screen film can have either single or double emulsion (sometimes referred to as *duplitized*). **Double-emulsion film** has emulsion coated on both sides of the base, and a layer of supercoat tops off each emulsion (Figure 6-5, *A*). General radiographic imaging typically uses a double-emulsion film with two intensifying screens.

  Single-emulsion screen film, with only one emulsion layer, is used with a single intensifying screen. It has many uses, including duplication, subtraction, computed tomography (CT), magnetic resonance imaging (MRI), sonography, nuclear medicine, mammography, and laser printing. Single-emulsion film is most different from double-emulsion film in that it contains an anticurl/antihalation layer (Figure 6-5, *B*).

  The anticurl/antihalation layer is a colored backing on single-emulsion film that prevents film from curling and prevents halation. *Halation* refers to an image

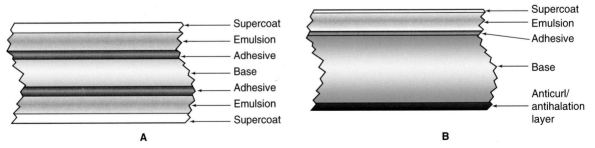

FIGURE 6-5 Cross-section of double-emulsion **(A)** and single-emulsion **(B)** film.

being recorded on the film by light that has been reflected back to expose the emulsion a second time. This light is that which would come from an intensifying screen as used in mammography; from the light source that is used in multiformat cameras used in CT, MRI, nuclear medicine, or sonography; or from the light source used in radiographic duplicators and subtractors. The dull side of single-emulsion film is the emulsion side, and the shiny side is the anticurl/antihalation side. This colored backing is removed during normal processing.

FILM CHARACTERISTICS

Current medical imaging film manufacturers offer a wide variety of films, differing not only in size and general type but also in respect to film speed, film contrast, exposure latitude, spectral sensitivity, and crossover.

Film Speed, Film Contrast, and Exposure Latitude

Two primary factors affect the sensitivity or **speed** of radiographic film. Both of these factors deal with the silver halide crystals that are found in the emulsion layer(s) of film. The first factor deals with the number of silver halide crystals present, and the second factor deals with the size of these silver halide crystals. Radiographic film manufacturers manipulate film speed by manipulating both of these factors in the production of specific speeds of radiographic film.

Important Relationship

Silver Halide and Film Sensitivity

As the number of silver halide crystals increases, film sensitivity or speed increases; as the size of the silver halide crystals increases, film sensitivity or speed increases.

Film contrast refers to the ability of radiographic film to provide a certain level of image contrast. High-contrast film demonstrates more black and white areas, whereas low-contrast film primarily shows shades of gray. Exposure latitude is closely related to film contrast.

Film speed, contrast, and latitude are graphically demonstrated in a film's characteristic (sensitometric) curve. Sensitometry is the study of the relationship between radiation exposure and the amount of density produced. This information is displayed as a curve on a graph (Figure 6-6), and every film has a different curve. Film sensitometry is discussed in greater detail in Chapter 8.

Spectral Sensitivity

Spectral sensitivity refers to the color of light to which a particular film is most sensitive. In radiography two categories of spectral sensitivity generally exist: blue-sensitive

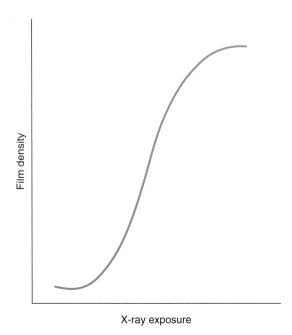

FIGURE 6-6 The characteristic (sensitometric) curve graphically represents the relationship between varying x-ray exposure and film density.

film and green-sensitive (orthochromatic) film. When radiographic film with intensifying screens is used, it is important to match the spectral sensitivity of the film with the spectral emission of the screens. **Spectral emission** refers to the color of light produced by a particular intensifying screen. In radiography two categories of spectral emission generally exist: blue light–emitting screens and green light–emitting screens. It is critical to use blue-sensitive film with blue light–emitting screens and green-sensitive film with green light–emitting screens. **Spectral matching** refers to correctly matching the color sensitivity of the film to the color emission of the intensifying screen. Making an incorrect match of film and screens based on spectral emission and sensitivity results in radiographs that display inappropriate levels of radiographic density.

Important Relationship

Spectral Matching and Density

To best use a film-screen system, the radiographer must match the color sensitivity of the film with the color emission of the intensifying screen. Failure to do so results in suboptimal density.

Spectral sensitivity also relates to the color of light produced with safelight filters. In the darkroom, safelight filters are placed in safelights to produce a particular color of light for illumination. It is important to use the appropriate safelight filter in all darkroom safelights based on the spectral sensitivity of the film being handled in that darkroom. The GBX filter is safe for both blue- and green-sensitive film. GBX simply stands for green/blue x-ray. The Wratten 1A safelight filter is safe for green-sensitive film only, and the Wratten 6B safelight filter is safe for blue-sensitive film only. Most laser film has to be handled in total darkness without any darkroom illumination whatsoever because of its sensitivity to the color light produced by safelight filters. Making an incorrect match between the type of safelight filter and the spectral sensitivity of film results in unusually high levels of safelight fogging on the film. This fogging appears radiographically as a film with increased density and decreased contrast.

Practical Tip

Spectral Emission and Spectral Sensitivity

The spectral emission of intensifying screens must be matched to the spectral sensitivity of the film. It is also important to make sure that the spectral emission of safelight filters in the darkroom is compatible with the spectral sensitivity of the film.

Crossover

Crossover is a problem that is unique to double-emulsion film used with intensifying screens. **Crossover** refers to light that has been produced by an intensifying screen exposing one emulsion and then crossing over the base layer of the film to expose the other emulsion (Figure 6-7, *A*). Crossover is a radiographic problem because it decreases recorded detail as seen on the image.

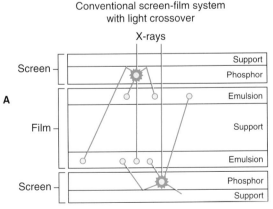

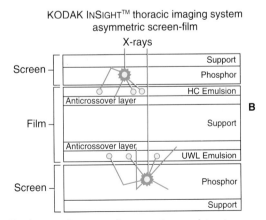

FIGURE 6-7 A, Light emitted from one screen crosses the film base and exposes the opposite emulsion in a conventional film-screen system. **B,** The asymmetric film-screen system has a faster back screen as well as a unique film that includes two different emulsions and zero-crossover or anticrossover technology. *Courtesy Eastman Kodak.*

Progress has been made in reducing crossover. The use of silver halide crystals created with the T-grain technology significantly lowers crossover. In addition, another recent innovation in double-emulsion film is referred to as *zero-crossover technology*. Adding an anticrossover layer on each side of the base layer next to each emulsion layer has essentially eliminated crossover.

Important Relationship

Crossover and Recorded Detail

When light from one intensifying screen crosses over the film base and exposes the emulsion on the opposite side, loss of recorded detail occurs. Reducing crossover improves recorded detail.

The Kodak InSight™ Thoracic Imaging System is an example of how zero-crossover technology is used (Figure 6-7, *B*). This system starts with a film with two different emulsions, one with relatively high film contrast and the other with low. This atypical film is combined with two very different intensifying screens, one much faster than the other (termed *asymmetric screens*). Zero-crossover layers ensure that the images form independently on each side of the base. The composite image produced with this system demonstrates lung detail as well as anatomy in the area of the mediastinum.

Intensifying Screens

PURPOSE AND FUNCTION

An **intensifying screen** is a device found in radiographic cassettes that contains phosphors that convert x-ray energy into light, which then exposes the radiographic film (Figure 6-8). A **phosphor** is a chemical compound that emits visible light when struck by radiation. The purpose of intensifying screens is to decrease the radiation dose to the patient. This decrease in radiation dose is in comparison to using an image receptor that does not use intensifying screens, as is the case with direct-exposure radiography. With direct-exposure radiography, only the transmitted x-rays produce the image of the body part. The film is simply placed inside a light-tight holder and then used as the image receptor. The addition of intensifying screens allows the radiographer to use significantly less mAs (the product of milliamperage and exposure time) than when not using screens, decreasing the patient dose and allowing shorter exposure times to be used. The primary trade-off or disadvantage to using intensifying screens is the reduction of recorded detail in the radiographic image.

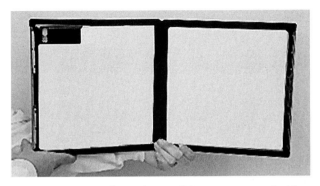

FIGURE 6-8 A typical set of intensifying screens seen inside a cassette. *From* Mosby's radiographic instructional series: radiographic imaging, *St Louis, 1998, Mosby.*

Important Relationship

Screens, Patient Exposure, and Recorded Detail

Compared with direct-exposure radiography, adding intensifying screens reduces patient exposure but also reduces recorded detail.

Intensifying screens intensify or amplify the amount of energy to which they are exposed. Without screens, the total amount of energy that the film is exposed to consists of x-rays. With screens, the total amount of energy that the film is exposed to is divided between x-rays and light. When intensifying screens are used, about 90% to 99% of the total energy that the film is exposed to is light. The remaining 1% to 10% of the energy is x-rays.

LUMINESCENCE

Intensifying screens operate by a process known as *luminescence*. **Luminescence** is the emission of light from the screen when stimulated by radiation. Intensifying screens may luminesce in two ways. The desired type of luminescence in imaging is fluorescence. **Fluorescence** refers to the ability of phosphors to emit visible light only while exposed to x-rays. *Phosphorescence* is another term to describe screen light emission. **Phosphorescence** occurs when screen phosphors continue to emit light after the x-ray exposure has stopped. Phosphorescence is sometimes called *screen lag* or *afterglow;* this result is undesirable.

SCREEN CONSTRUCTION

As with radiographic film, the construction of screens can be described in layers (Figure 6-9). The outermost layer, found closest to the film, is the protective

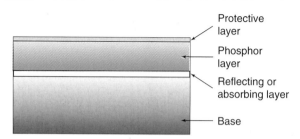

FIGURE 6-9 Cross-section of an intensifying screen.

layer. The **protective layer** is made of plastic and protects the fragile phosphor material underneath it. The **phosphor layer,** or active layer, is the most important screen component because it contains the phosphor material that absorbs the transmitted x-rays and converts them to visible light. Sometimes, a light-absorbing dye is added to the phosphor layer to decrease the total amount of light striking the film.

The next layer can be either a **reflecting layer** or an **absorbing layer.** Intensifying screens usually are manufactured with one or the other, but never with both. If a reflecting layer is present, it consists of either magnesium oxide or titanium dioxide. Because phosphors emit light in all directions, its purpose is to reflect light back toward the film. If an absorbing layer is used, it generally is a light-absorbing dye. The dye is used to absorb light emitted toward it by the phosphor layer.

The bottom layer of the intensifying screen, found farthest from the film, is the **base.** Made of polyester or cardboard, the base must be flexible and chemically stable. The base provides support and stability for the phosphor layer.

Intensifying screen systems used in cassettes generally include two screens. The screen that is mounted in the tube side of the cassette is called the *front screen,* and the screen that is mounted in the opposite side is called the *back screen.* With two screens, the film (double emulsion) is exposed to approximately twice as much light as in a single-screen system because the film is exposed to light from both sides. Some screen systems use only a single screen and are used with single-emulsion film. When only a single screen is used, it is mounted as a back screen on the side of the cassette that is opposite from the tube side.

SCREEN CHARACTERISTICS

Types of Phosphors

A large number of different phosphor materials are available for today's intensifying screens (Table 6-1). The most common phosphor material consists of some element from the rare earth group of elements. **Rare earth elements** are those that range in atomic number from 57 to 71 on the periodic table of the elements; they are referred to as *rare earth elements* because they are relatively difficult and expensive to extract from the earth. Rare earth phosphors have replaced calcium tungstate in the

TABLE 6-1   **INTENSIFYING SCREEN PHOSPHOR MATERIALS AND THEIR SPECTRAL EMISSIONS**

Phosphor	Spectral Emission
Calcium tungstate ($CaWO_4$)*	Blue
Rare earth elements	
Lanthanum oxybromide (LaOBr)	Blue
Yttrium tantalate ($YTaO_4$)	Ultraviolet/blue
Gadolinium oxysulfide (Gd_2O_2S)	Green
Others	
Barium lead sulfate ($BaPbSO_4$)	Blue
Barium strontium sulfate ($BaSrSO_4$)	Blue

*No longer manufactured but may be in limited use.

modern practice of radiography. Calcium tungstate was the mainstay phosphor used in intensifying screens until the 1970s. At that time, research revealed that, compared with calcium tungstate, rare earth phosphors absorb more x-rays, convert the x-rays to visible light more efficiently, and result in improved recorded detail in the radiographic image. For these reasons, rare earth phosphors have effectively replaced calcium tungstate in today's intensifying screens.

Intensifying screen phosphors can be differentiated based on the color of visible light they emit, or their spectral emission. Calcium tungstate phosphors produce light in the blue region of the spectrum, whereas rare earth phosphors may produce green or blue light depending on the phosphor (see Table 6-1). Because film emulsion is developed to be sensitive to a specific color of light, it is extremely important that the film and screen be matched appropriately. *Spectral matching* refers to using blue-sensitive film with blue light–emitting screens and likewise green-sensitive (orthochromatic) film with screens that emit green light. Failure to match the screen and film results in inappropriate radiographic density.

Screen Speed

The purpose of intensifying screens is to decrease the radiation dose to the patient. Because screen phosphors can intensify the action of the x-rays by converting them to visible light, the use of screens allows the radiographer to use considerably less mAs than that required with direct-exposure radiography. In addition, it is important to remember that the drawback to using screens is the reduction in recorded detail. Screen manufacturers produce a variety of intensifying screens, differing in how well they intensify the action of the x-rays as well as in their capacity to produce accurate recorded detail.

The capability of a screen to produce visible light is called **screen speed,** with a faster screen producing more light than a slower screen (given the same exposure). Screen speed can be identified in a number of ways, including the intensification factor and relative screen speed.

Important Relationship

Screen Speed and Light Emission

The faster an intensifying screen, the more light emitted for the same x-ray exposure.

The intensifying action of screens can be described by a formula, the intensification factor. This factor accurately represents the degree to which exposure factors (and patient dose) are reduced when intensifying screens are used. The **intensification factor (IF)** can be stated as follows:

$$IF = \frac{\text{Exposure required without screens}}{\text{Exposure required with screens}}$$

X *Mathematical Application*

The Intensification Factor

If a radiograph of a hand was produced with 100 mAs using direct exposure and a radiograph of the same hand was produced with an intensifying screen system using 4 mAs, resulting in the same density as the first film, what is the IF of the screen system?

$$IF = \frac{100 \text{ mAs}}{4 \text{ mAs}}$$

$$IF = 25$$

This indicates that 25 times the exposure would be needed to produce a radiograph with comparable density if a direct-exposure system was used.

Important Relationship

Screen Speed and Patient Dose

As screen speed increases, radiation dose to the patient decreases; as screen speed decreases, radiation dose to the patient increases.

The ability of the screen to produce visible light, and therefore density, can also be described in terms of its **relative speed.** Relative speed results from comparing screen-film systems based on the amount of light (and density) produced for a given exposure. The amount of light produced with a par (or medium) speed calcium tungstate screen system is used as the standard for comparison and is assigned a relative speed of 100. Given the same exposure, a 200 speed system is able to produce twice as much light (and density), whereas a 400 speed system will produce four times as much light as the system using a par speed calcium tungstate screen.

Important Relationship

Screen Speed and Density

As screen speed increases, density increases; as screen speed decreases, density decreases.

The mathematical relationship between screen speed and density is directly proportionate. The **mAs conversion formula for screens** is a formula that is helpful for the radiographer to use in determining how to compensate or adjust mAs when changing intensifying screen system speeds. This formula is stated as follows:

$$\frac{mAs_1}{mAs_2} = \frac{\text{Relative screen speed}_2}{\text{Relative screen speed}_1}$$

X Mathematical Application

Use of the mAs Conversion Formula for Screens

If 10 mAs were used with a 400 speed screen system to produce an optimal radiograph, what mAs would be necessary to produce a radiograph with the same density using a 100 speed screen system?

$$\frac{10 \text{ mAs}}{mAs_2} = \frac{100 \text{ relative speed}}{400 \text{ relative speed}}$$

$$mAs_2 = 40$$

Factors Affecting Screen Speed

Most radiology departments use at least two different speeds of intensifying screen systems. A fast system usually is available with a relative speed of about 400. A 400 speed system is a good compromise between the beneficial effect of decreasing the patient dose and the detrimental effect of decreasing the recorded detail. This system should be used for radiographic procedures of the thorax, abdomen, pelvis, skull, and facial bones (excluding the mandible and nasal bones), as well as for examinations requiring the use of a contrast medium. A slower system is usually available also, and it is sometimes labeled on the outside of the cassette as "detail" or "extremity." The relative speed of this system typically is about 100. This system should be used when radiographing the extremities, mandible, and nasal bones, studies that do not require the use of a grid. Detail or extremity screen systems are relatively slow, thereby requiring greater exposure and resulting in higher patient doses. However, the anatomic parts imaged with detail or extremity screen systems generally are small, therefore not requiring large exposures. Detail or extremity screen systems produce excellent recorded detail. The radiographer must be careful in selecting the appropriate screen system for the examination ordered.

 Practical Tip

Selecting a Screen Speed

The radiographer should select the film-screen system that will balance patient exposure and recorded detail.

Several factors affect how fast or slow an intensifying screen will be, including absorption efficiency, conversion efficiency, thickness of the phosphor layer, and size of the phosphor crystal. Also, the presence of a reflecting layer, an absorbing layer, or dye in the phosphor layer will affect screen speed.

Differences in absorption and conversion efficiency have played a large part in the switch from calcium tungstate to rare earth phosphor screens. *Absorption efficiency* refers to the screen's ability to absorb the incident x-ray photons. A rare earth phosphor screen absorbs approximately 60% of the incident photons, compared with calcium tungstate, which absorbs about 30% to 40%. Mathematically, this means that if 100 x-ray photons were to interact with these screens, the rare earth screen would absorb about 60 photons and the calcium tungstate 35. *Conversion efficiency* has to do with how well the screen phosphor takes these x-ray photons and converts them to visible light. Once again, the rare earth phosphors are superior. Rare earth phosphors produce three to four times the amount of visible light per absorbed photon than does calcium tungstate. The increased absorption and conversion efficiency mean that rare earth phosphors are significantly faster than calcium tungstate. This increased speed results in the radiographer being able to substantially reduce the x-ray exposure needed to produce images with the appropriate amount of density.

 Important Relationship

Rare Earth Phosphors and Speed

Rare earth phosphors are significantly faster than calcium tungstate because of increased absorption and conversion efficiency.

Because of the high absorption efficiency of rare earth phosphors, some screen manufacturers have developed cassettes that have asymmetric screens, or screens that are not identical. With asymmetric screens, the back screen is faster than the front, compensating for the reduction of x-ray photons that were absorbed by the front screen. In this situation, having a faster back screen will equalize the light exposure to both sides of the film emulsion.

For both calcium tungstate and rare earth phosphors, the thickness of the phosphor layer and the size of the crystal also have an impact on screen speed. A thicker phosphor layer contains more phosphor material than a thinner phosphor layer. Because the phosphor is the material that converts x-rays into light, if more phosphor material is present in a screen, more light will be produced, increasing the screen speed. The size of the phosphor material crystal also affects screen speed. A larger phosphor crystal produces more light than a smaller phosphor crystal. Again, more light being produced means that the screen is faster.

Important Relationship

Phosphor Thickness, Crystal Size, and Screen Speed

As the thickness of the phosphor layer increases, the speed of the intensifying screen increases; as the size of the phosphor crystals increases, the speed of the screen increases.

The final factors that affect screen speed are the presence or absence of a reflecting layer, a light-absorbing layer, or light-absorbing dyes in the phosphor layer. A reflecting layer is used to increase screen speed by reflecting light back toward the film (Figure 6-10). A light-absorbing layer or light-absorbing dyes present in the phosphor layer are used to decrease screen speed by absorbing light that would otherwise reach and expose the film.

Screen Speed and Recorded Detail

As stated earlier, the purpose of using intensifying screens rather than direct exposure is to decrease patient dose. Screens accomplish this purpose very well but at the expense of recorded detail.

When a phosphor crystal is energized by an x-ray photon, light is emitted from the crystal and spreads out toward the film emulsion. The actual physical area of the film exposed to light from a single phosphor crystal is greater than the area of film that would be exposed by an x-ray photon (Figure 6-11). This spreading out of the radiographic information decreases the recorded detail of that image, creating more image unsharpness. Light that originates from larger crystals or farther from the film emulsion (with a thicker phosphor layer) will have more spread, resulting in an even greater loss of recorded detail.

The presence or absence of a reflecting layer, an absorbing layer, or light-absorbing dyes also affects recorded detail. Because reflecting layers cause the light

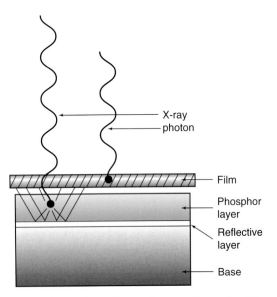

FIGURE 6-10 The reflecting layer redirects the visible light emitted by the screen phosphor toward the film emulsion. This process increases the speed of the screen but also results in a loss of recorded detail.

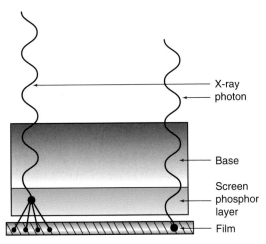

FIGURE 6-11 In comparison with the x-ray photon that directly exposes the film, the x-ray photon that interacts with the intensifying screen produces visible light. Before the film is exposed, the light spreads out, resulting in a loss of recorded detail.

TABLE 6-2	SUMMARY OF EFFECT OF SCREEN FACTORS ON SCREEN SPEED, RECORDED DETAIL, AND PATIENT DOSE		
Screen Factor	**Screen Speed**	**Recorded Detail**	**Patient Dose**
Thicker phosphor layer	↑	↓	↓
Larger phosphor crystal size	↑	↓	↓
Reflective layer	↑	↓	↓
Absorbing layer	↓	↑	↑
Dye in phosphor layer	↓	↑	↑

photons to travel farther and spread out more, screens with reflecting layers decrease recorded detail. Screens with absorbing layers or light-absorbing dyes that have been added to the phosphor layers reduce the speed of the screen and, by absorbing the lower-energy light photons, improve the level of recorded detail. The effect of these screen construction factors on screen speed, recorded detail, and patient dose are summarized in Table 6-2.

Screen Speed and Recorded Detail

With any given phosphor type, as screen speed increases, recorded detail decreases, and as screen speed decreases, recorded detail increases.

The phosphor material, being either a rare earth element or calcium tungstate, affects recorded detail. Although it seems paradoxical, film-screen systems that use rare earth phosphors produce greater recorded detail than calcium tungstate systems. In that rare earth phosphors are so much more efficient at absorbing the x-ray photons and converting them to light, it is possible to have a very fast system with a screen that has a thin phosphor layer and/or small crystals. It is also possible to use a slower speed film with rare earth screens, to maintain an increase in relative speed compared with calcium tungstate, and to provide improved recorded detail. This is why rare earth screens have become so popular. They are faster than calcium tungstate and produce better recorded detail as well.

Quantum Mottle

Quantum mottle, commonly called *image noise*, can be defined as the statistical fluctuation in the quantity of x-ray photons that contribute to image formation per square millimeter. When a very low number of photons are needed by the intensifying screens to produce appropriate image density, the image will appear mottled, or splotchy. This appearance can also be described as a "salt and pepper look," as compared with a consistent, homogenous density. This is often a direct result of using very fast speed film-screen systems, which require very small amounts of exposure. Quantum mottle decreases recorded detail, resulting in a radiographic image that is grainy in appearance (Figure 6-12, *A*). An optimal image displays more recorded detail (Figure 6-12, *B*). The only strategy for reducing quantum mottle is the use of more mAs (more photons). Using a slower speed system or adjusting the mAs and kilovoltage peak can alleviate image noise or quantum mottle.

SCREEN MAINTENANCE

The maintenance of intensifying screens is significant because radiographic quality depends in large part on how well the screens are continuously maintained. Two important maintenance procedures should be performed on intensifying screens. One of these is regular cleaning. The outside surface of screens come into contact with the environment and with the hands of those who are unloading and loading cassettes, resulting in the natural oils on fingers and hands being deposited on the screen surface. These oils tend to attract dust and dirt, which can build up to the point that they are actually imaged on radiographs as artifacts. Screen cleaning

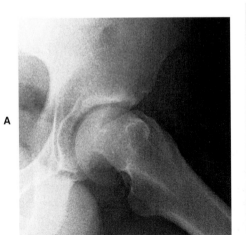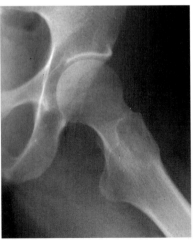

FIGURE 6-12 **A,** This hip radiograph demonstrates the mottled, grainy appearance associated with quantum mottle resulting from a low number of x-ray photons being used to produce the image. **B,** In comparison, an optimal hip image shows greater recorded detail.

should be done routinely. The cleaning is accomplished with commercially available antistatic intensifying screen cleaner fluid and gauze pads.

Another important maintenance procedure it to check cassettes for film screen contact. Good **film-screen contact** exists when the screen or screens are in intimate contact with the film. Poor film-screen contact greatly degrades recorded detail and is usually seen as a localized area of unsharpness somewhere on the radiographic image. Rarely is film-screen contact so poor that unsharpness can be seen across the entire radiograph. A major part of testing for film-screen contact is identifying problem cassettes.

 Practical Tip

Identifying Cassettes

When it is necessary to find the specific cassette that has a problem, it can be done easily by numbering the cassettes. An excellent way to accomplish this is to write the cassette number (using a permanent black marker) on the surface of one of the screens in a corner out of the way. That same number then needs to be written on the outside of the cassette. The screen number will show up on images produced with that cassette, and if there is a problem, knowing this number will allow the radiographer to find and test the cassette in question.

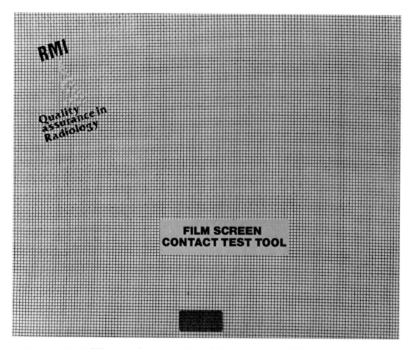

FIGURE 6-13 Wire mesh test tool used for evaluating film-screen contact.

The film-screen contact test is easily accomplished, but it requires a special wire mesh test tool (Figure 6-13). The wire mesh tool is simply placed on the cassette in question and radiographed at an appropriate technique. The resultant radiograph (Figure 6-14) is then viewed at a distance of about 6 feet to determine whether there are any areas of unsharpness, indicating poor recorded detail. Areas of poor contact will appear darker than areas of good contact because of the increased spreading out of the light photons. This test should be done every 6 months or annually.

Cassettes

The remaining component in the conventional image receptor is the cassette (Figure 6-15). Serving as a container for both the intensifying screens and the film, the cassette must be light-proof, weigh little enough to be portable, and be rigid enough not to bend under a patient's weight, all while allowing the maximum amount of radiation to pass through and reach the screens. Low x-ray–absorbing materials, such as Bakelite, magnesium, or even graphite carbon, can be found in the front of cassettes. Inside the back of cassettes, there may be a thin sheet of lead foil, designed to absorb backscatter before it exposes the film. Finally, cassettes must be constructed in such a way as to maintain good film-screen contact.

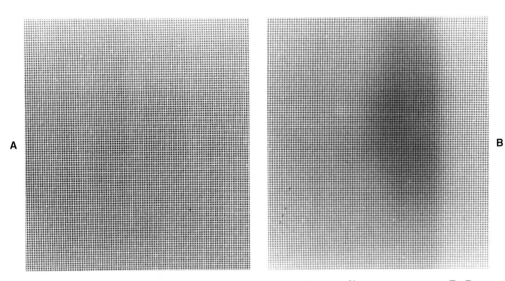

A   **B**

FIGURE 6-14 Images produced with wire mesh test. **A,** Proper film-screen contact. **B,** Poor film-screen contact. *From Bushong S: Radiographic science for technologists, ed 6, St Louis, 1997, Mosby.*

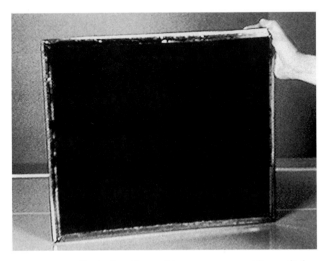

FIGURE 6-15 Typical radiographic cassette, providing a light-proof container for intensifying screens and film. *From Mosby's radiographic instructional series: radiographic imaging, St Louis, 1998, Mosby.*

FILM CRITIQUE

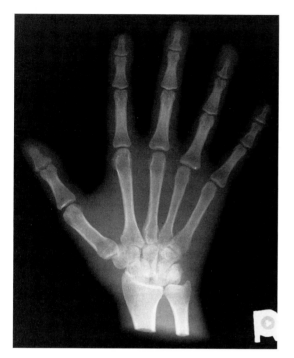

FIGURE 6-16 Image A was produced using 57 kVp, 50 mA at 0.040 s, 100 speed film-screen combination, and a 40-inch source-to-image receptor distance.

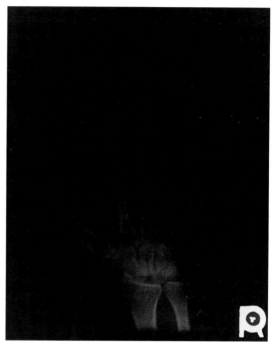

FIGURE 6-17 Image B was produced using 57 kVp, 160 mA at 0.0125 s, 400 speed film-screen combination, and a 40-inch source-to-image receptor distance.

1. Evaluate each radiograph and discuss its quality.

2. For each image, evaluate the exposure variables and discuss their effect on the quality of the image, regardless of whether it is apparent on the radiograph.

3. For each image, identify any adjustments that could be made in the exposure factors to produce an optimal image.

Review Questions

1. The radiation- and light-sensitive layer of radiographic film is the _____ layer.
   A. base
   B. emulsion
   C. supercoat
   D. anticurl/antihalation

2. Crossover is a radiographic problem because it decreases
   A. contrast.
   B. density.
   C. recorded detail.
   D. film speed.

3. Spectral sensitivity refers to the color sensitivity of
   A. radiographic film.
   B. safelight filters.
   C. intensifying screens.
   D. safelight filters and intensifying screens.

4. During latent image formation, electrons that have been liberated by radiation or light exposure are attracted to the
   A. bromide.
   B. sensitivity specks.
   C. bound silver ions.
   D. gelatin.

5. Silver halide crystals are found in the
   A. film base.
   B. supercoat.
   C. emulsion.
   D. anticurl/antihalation layer.

6. Which of the following is the most common type of film for general radiographic examinations?
   A. Direct exposure
   B. Screen, single emulsion
   C. Screen, double emulsion
   D. Rare earth

7. Poor film-screen contact results in a loss of
   A. density.
   B. contrast.
   C. recorded detail.
   D. speed.

8. The purpose of intensifying screens is to
   A. increase radiographic density.
   B. increase recorded detail.
   C. decrease recorded detail.
   D. decrease patient dose.

9. The most common phosphor material used in today's intensifying screens is
   A. calcium tungstate.
   B. rare earth elements.
   C. silver halide.
   D. barium sulfate.

10. The speed of an intensifying screen can be reduced by adding
    A. more phosphor.
    B. a reflecting layer.
    C. larger phosphor crystals.
    D. dye to the phosphor layer.

11. What is the intensification factor for screens that require 5 mAs to produce the same density as produced by direct exposure using 150 mAs?
  A. 5
  B. 30
  C. 50
  D. 300

12. If 25 mAs is used with a 500 speed film-screen system to produce an optimal image, how much mAs is needed to produce the same density with 100 speed system?
  A. 5 mAs
  B. 100 mAs
  C. 125 mAs
  D. 300 mAs

13. Typically, as screen speed decreases, _____ decreases.
  A. density
  B. recorded detail
  C. patient dose
  D. x-ray exposure

14. Which of the following strategies will help reduce quantum mottle?
  A. Using a faster speed film-screen system
  B. Increasing kilovoltage peak and reducing mAs
  C. Reducing kilovoltage peak and increasing mAs
  D. Reducing kilovoltage peak and reducing mAs

15. The wire mesh test tool is used to evaluate
  A. screen speed.
  B. screen resolution.
  C. screen cleanliness.
  D. film-screen contact.

CHAPTER 7

Radiographic Processing

PURPOSE

AUTOMATIC PROCESSING EQUIPMENT

PROCESSING STAGES

Developing
Fixing
Drying

PROCESSING SYSTEMS

Tanks
Vertical Transport System
Motor Drive
Replenishment System
Recirculation System
Temperature Control
Drying System

INADEQUATE PROCESSING

FILM-HANDLING AREAS

Storing Unexposed Film
Storing Radiographs
The Darkroom

PROCESSING QUALITY CONTROL

SILVER RECOVERY

RADIOGRAPHIC ARTIFACTS

REVIEW QUESTIONS

1 Define all of the key terms in this chapter.

2 State all of the important relationships in this chapter.

3 State the purpose of radiographic processing.

4 Describe the various processing stages, systems, and rollers.

5 List the developing and fixing solution agents and state their function.

6 Discuss the role of developer temperature in processing.

7 Describe the washing and drying processing stages.

8 List problems of inadequate processing and their radiographic presentation.

9 State the importance of replenishment during processing.

10 List important considerations in the handling and storage of film before and after processing.

11 Describe the importance of darkroom design.

12 State the importance of and process of silver recovery.

13 Recognize radiographic artifacts and their causes.

KEY TERMS

latent image
manifest image
automatic processor
processing cycle
processor capacity
developing, or reducing, agents
superadditivity
accelerator/activator agent
restrainer
preservative (developer)
hardener (developer)
solvent
fixing agent
acidifier
preservative (fixer)
hardener (fixer)
diffusion

feedtray
entrance roller assembly
transport rollers
turnaround roller
crossover roller
guide plates
standby control
replenishment
aerial oxidation
use oxidation
flood replenishment
recirculation system
immersion heater
FIFO
silver recovery
artifact

Processing converts an invisible image on exposed film into a permanent visible radiographic image. Automatic processing equipment consists of a series of tanks, rollers, systems, and processing stages. The stages of development and fixation use a combination of chemicals that interact with the film emulsion(s) to produce the visible image.

Considerations in film handling, darkroom design, and silver recovery are also important to the overall quality of radiographs and environmental health. In addition, the prevention of radiographic artifacts is necessary for the overall production of a quality radiograph.

Purpose

The purpose of radiographic processing is to convert the latent image into a manifest image. The **latent image** is that image that exists on the film after exposure but before processing. The **manifest image** is that image that exists on the film after processing.

The electrochemical process that occurs according to the Gurney-Mott theory is the first step toward creating a visible image on radiographic film. Exposure of the silver bromide crystal in the film emulsion by light or x-ray photons initiates an electrochemical process (Figure 7-1). Chemical processing of the exposed film completes the conversion process and transforms the image into a permanent visible image.

Automatic Processing Equipment

An **automatic processor** (Figure 7-2) is a device that encompasses chemical tanks, a roller transport system, and a dryer system for the processing of radiographic film. Many manufacturers produce automatic processors and many models of this type of equipment. Different models of automatic processors vary in terms of processing cycle and processor capacity. **Processing cycle** refers to the amount of time it takes to process a single piece of film. This amount of time varies among processors, between 45 seconds and 3.5 minutes. **Processor capacity** refers to the number of films that can be processed per hour. Processor capacity depends on the film size and can be expressed in terms of the number of films of equal size processed in 1 hour, or it can be expressed in terms of the number of films of multiple sizes processed in 1 hour. It is important to know the processing cycle and capacity of a processor when purchasing one.

Processing Stages

The processing of a radiograph occurs in four stages: developing, fixing, washing, and drying. Each stage has its specific function and processing method.

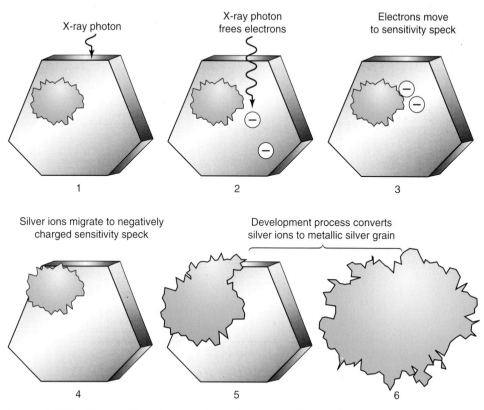

FIGURE 7-1 The Gurney-Mott theory explains the process of converting the exposed silver bromide crystals to black metallic silver. Chemical development continues this process and completes the conversion. (Numbers indicate steps in the process.)

DEVELOPING

The primary function of developing is to convert the latent image into a manifest or visible image. There are also two secondary purposes of developing. One is to amplify the amount of metallic silver on the film by increasing the number of silver atoms in each latent image center. The other is to reduce the exposed silver halide crystals into metallic silver.

During the development process, developer solution donates additional electrons to the sensitivity specks, or electron traps, in the emulsion layer(s) of the film. These additional electrons attract more silver to these areas, thereby amplifying the amount of atomic silver at each latent image center. Exposed silver halide is reduced to metallic silver by removing bromide and iodide ions from the emulsion. The atomic silver that was exposed to radiant energy (light and x-rays) is converted to metallic silver and demonstrated as radiographic densities. Unexposed silver halide will not react immediately to developer because it has not been ionized and will

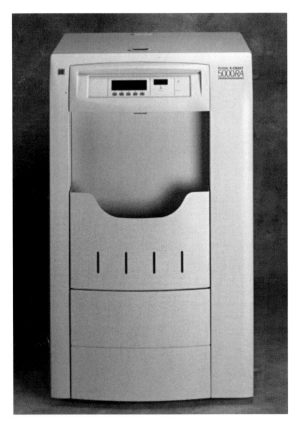

FIGURE 7-2 A type of automatic processor used in radiography. *Courtesy Eastman Kodak Company.*

not accept electrons from the developer. Given extended exposure to developing solution or exposure to excessively heated developing solution, however, even unexposed areas of film can react to developing solution. Exposed silver halide reacts to developer by accepting electrons because neutral atomic silver that was previously bonded to either bromide or iodide has room to accept electrons in its outer-most electron shell (the O-shell).

Developing, or Reducing, Agents

The purpose of the **developing,** or **reducing, agents** is to reduce exposed silver halide to metallic silver and to add electrons to exposed silver halide. Two chemicals are used to accomplish this purpose: phenidone and hydroquinone. Phenidone is said to be a fast reducer, producing gray (lower) densities. Hydroquinone is said to be a slow reducer, producing black (higher) densities.

Producing Radiographic Densities

The developing agents are responsible for reducing the exposed silver halide crystals to metallic silver, visualized as optical densities. Phenidone is responsible for creating the lower densities, and hydroquinone is responsible for creating the higher densities. Their combined effect results in the range of visible densities on the radiograph.

Both phenidone and hydroquinone also act to soften and swell the emulsion(s). Phenidone and hydroquinone are said to be synergistic, or to have superadditivity. **Superadditivity** means that together these chemicals produce a greater effect on the film than they would individually. This is used to advantage by using both chemicals in combination to develop or reduce the exposed silver halide.

Accelerator, or Activator, Agent

The purpose of the **accelerator, or activator, agent** (sometimes also called a *buffering agent*) is to elevate and maintain the pH of the developer solution. The pH measures the alkalinity of the solution that is needed for the reducing agents. A loss of pH means a loss of developer activity. A carbonate, such as sodium carbonate, is the chemical used as this agent.

Restrainer

The purpose of the **restrainer** is to decrease the reduction or development of unexposed silver halide. Such reduction or development is generally referred to as *chemical fog* because some chemicals (usually the reducing agents) can create densities in areas of the film where no densities should be present. A bromide, such as potassium bromide, is the chemical used as this agent.

Preservative

The purpose of the **preservative** is to decrease oxidation of the developer solution. Oxidation acts to decrease the chemical activity of developer that begins almost immediately after the developer solution is mixed. A sulfite, such as sodium sulfite, is the chemical used as this agent.

Hardener

The purpose of the **hardener** is to harden the emulsion that was softened by the reducing or developing agents. This hardening process protects the radiographic image present on the film from being damaged from the roller transport system. Glutaraldehyde is the chemical used as the hardener.

Solvent

The purpose of the **solvent** is to dilute the chemicals in the developer solution, which causes these chemicals to function at their desired level of activity. The solvent is simply water. Developer chemicals are available in liquid form and generally are packaged in three separate packages for mixing with water.

Each of these agents and their chemicals and functions are summarized in Table 7-1.

FIXING

The primary functions of the fixing stage are to remove undeveloped silver halide from the film and to make the remaining image permanent. There are also two secondary functions of fixing. One is to stop the development process; the other is to further harden the emulsion(s). Fixing solution must function to remove all undeveloped silver halide while not affecting the metallic silver image.

Fixing Agent

The purpose of the **fixing agent** is to clear undeveloped silver halide away from the film. A thiosulfate (sometimes also called *hypo*), such as ammonium thiosulfate, is the chemical used as this agent.

TABLE 7-1	DEVELOPER SOLUTION AGENTS, CHEMICALS, AND THEIR FUNCTIONS	
Agent	**Chemical(s)**	**Function**
Developing or reducing agents	Phenidone	Fast-reducing, produces gray densities
	Hydroquinone	Slow-reducing, produces black densities
Accelerator or activator	Sodium carbonate	Elevates and maintains solution pH
Restrainer	Potassium bromide	Decreases reduction of unexposed silver halide
Preservative	Sodium sulfite	Decreases oxidation of solution
Hardener	Glutaraldehyde	Hardens the emulsion(s)
Solvent	Water	Dilutes the chemicals

> ### Important Relationship
>
> *Clearing the Unexposed Crystals*
>
> The fixing agent, ammonium thiosulfate, is responsible for removing the unexposed crystals from the emulsion.

Acidifier

The purpose of the **acidifier** (sometimes called a *buffer*) is to stop the development process and create an acid pH environment for the fixing agent. An acid, such as acetic acid, is the chemical used as this agent.

Preservative

The purposes of the **preservative** are to protect the fixing agent from oxidation and to maintain its activity level. Oxidization and developer carryover can decrease the strength of the fixing agent. A sulfite, such as sodium sulfite, is the chemical used as this agent.

Hardener

The purpose of the **hardener** is to further harden the emulsion to make the resultant manifest image permanent for handling. An aluminum salt, such as chrome alum, potassium alum, aluminum sulfate, or aluminum chloride, is the chemical used as this agent.

Solvent

The purpose of the solvent is to dilute the chemicals in the fixer solution so that the chemicals can function at their desired level of activity. The solvent is simply water. Fixer chemicals are available in liquid form and generally are packaged in two separate packages for mixing with water.

Each of these agents and their chemicals and functions are summarized in Table 7-2.

Washing

The purpose of the washing process is to remove fixing solution from the surface of the film. This is a further step in making the manifest image permanent. If not properly washed, the resulting radiograph will show a brown staining of the image, resulting in image loss and a decrease in its diagnostic value. This staining is caused by thiosulfate (fixing agent) that remains in the emulsion(s). Some thiosulfate will always remain within the film, but the goal of washing is to remove enough so that the radiograph will be usable for an extended period.

TABLE 7-2   FIXER SOLUTION AGENTS, CHEMICALS, AND THEIR FUNCTIONS

Agent	Chemical(s)	Function
Fixing agent	Ammonium thiosulfate	Clears away undeveloped silver halide
Acidifier	Acetic acid	Stops development
Preservative	Sodium sulfite	Prevents reaction between fixing agent and acidifier
Hardener	Chrome alum, potassium alum, aluminum sulfate, or aluminum chloride	Hardens the emulsion

Important Relationship

Archival Quality of Radiographs

Maintaining the archival (long-term) quality of radiographs requires that most of the fixing agent be removed (washed) from the film. Staining or fading of the permanent image results when too much thiosulfate remains on the film.

The process by which washing works is referred to as *diffusion*. **Diffusion** works by exposing the film to water that contains less thiosulfate than the film does. Because the film contains more fixing agent than the water, the fixing agent diffuses into the water.

Eventually, thiosulfate concentrations in the wash water can become greater than those in the films that are being processed; therefore the wash water must be replaced frequently. The wash tank does not use the same replenishment system as the developer and fixer tanks. Instead, water flows freely from the input water supply through the wash tank and down the drain while the roller transport system is operating. This type of system provides a constant supply of fresh wash water to aid in the diffusion process. The moving water also causes agitation and increases diffusion.

DRYING

The final process in automatic processing is drying. The purpose of drying films is to remove 85% to 90% of the moisture from the film so that it can be handled easily and stored while maintaining the quality of the diagnostic image. As a result, finished radiographs should retain 10% to 15% of their moisture when processing is complete. If films are dried excessively, emulsion(s) can crack, decreasing the diagnostic quality of the radiograph.

Permanent radiographs must retain moisture of 10% to 15% to maintain archival quality. Excessive drying can cause the emulsion(s) to crack.

Increased relative humidity decreases the efficiency of dryers in processors, so an increased drying temperature is necessary. Processors are equipped with thermostatic controls to allow a wide range of dryer temperatures to be selected. For this chemical process to occur, specialized equipment, components, and systems must perform concurrently to move the film through the processing stages according to the manufacturer's specifications.

Processing Systems

TANKS

An automatic processor has three tanks: one for developer solution, one for fixer solution, and a wash tank for water. These tanks are made of stainless steel to prevent corrosion, and they provide a surface that is cleaned easily. The developer tank is the deepest, followed by the fixer tank, and then the wash tank. Considering that a film moves through the processor at a constant speed, it spends most of the time in the developer tank, somewhat less time in the fixer tank, and the least amount time in the wash tank.

VERTICAL TRANSPORT SYSTEM

Automatic processors use a vertical transport system of rollers that transport the film through the various stages of film processing (Figure 7-3). All rollers in a processor move at the same speed. A film is introduced into the processor on the feedtray (Figure 7-4). The **feedtray** is a flat metal surface with an edge on either side that permits the film to enter the processor easily and in a straight orientation. As the film enters the processor from the feedtray, the first roller assembly that it encounters is the entrance roller assembly. The **entrance roller assembly** consists of rollers that are covered with corrugated rubber (Figure 7-5). These corrugations assist in straightening out the path of the film so that it moves through the processor efficiently. Once a piece of film has moved through the roller assembly, an audible signal is given as an indication that it is safe to insert another piece of film into the processor. Ignoring this signal by inserting a piece of film too close behind another one will cause the films to overlap. Overlapping films can cause the transport roller system to jam or cause inadequate processing of both films.

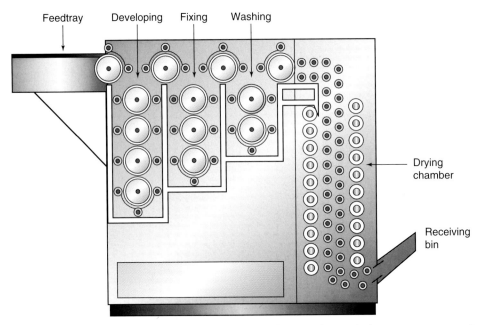

FIGURE 7-3 Cross-section of an automatic processor showing the vertical transport system of rollers.

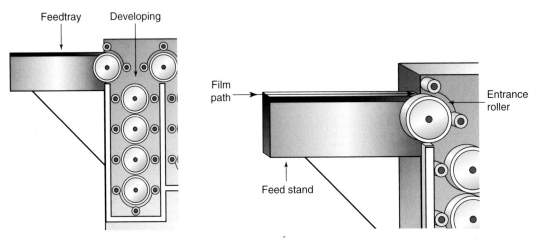

FIGURE 7-4 The feedtray permits the film to enter the processor easily and in a straight orientation.

FIGURE 7-5 The entrance roller assembly assists in straightening out the path of the film so that it moves through the processor efficiently.

The next type of roller that the film encounters is a transport roller (Figure 7-6). **Transport rollers** move the film through the chemical tanks and dryer assembly. Transport rollers are found on each side of a roller assembly. As the film enters a transport assembly, the transport rollers move the film down into the tank. The rollers also move the film up through the tank on the other side of the roller assembly. A

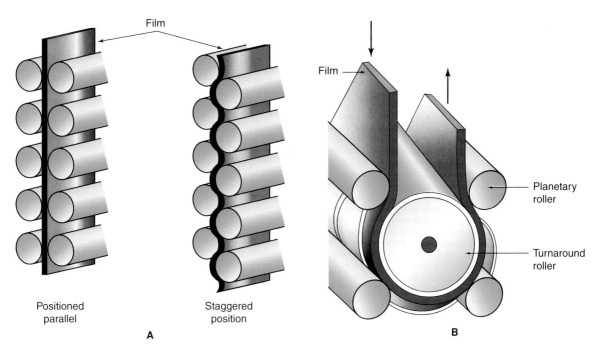

FIGURE 7-6 A, Transport rollers are positioned either parallel or staggered and move the film through the various stages of processing. **B,** Turnaround rollers at the bottom of the assembly turn the film from moving down to moving up.

turnaround roller at the bottom of the roller assembly turns the film from moving down the transport assembly to moving up. Transport rollers and turnaround rollers are often called *deep rollers* because they are immersed in liquid in the processor tanks.

The final type of roller used in the vertical transport system is the crossover roller (see Figure 7-6). The **crossover roller** assembly moves the film from one tank to another and into the dryer assembly. That is, crossover rollers cross the film from one transport assembly to another. Crossover rollers typically have a tight space between them to effect a squeegee-type action on the film. This squeegee effect assists in removing as much liquid from the film as can reasonably be accomplished before the film enters the next stage of processing, making that next stage of processing more efficient. There are crossover assemblies between each transport assembly in the processor (Figure 7-7).

In addition to the different roller assemblies that make up the vertical transport system, there are also guide plates on these roller assemblies. **Guide plates** are slightly curved metal plates that guide the leading edge of the moving film in a proper path through the roller assembly. Guide plates are located in several areas of the roller assemblies (Figure 7-8).

MOTOR DRIVE

An electric motor provides power for the roller assemblies to transport the film through the processor. An on/off switch that provides electrical power to the processor

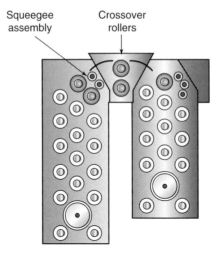

FIGURE 7-7 Crossover rollers are located between each transport assembly in the processor.

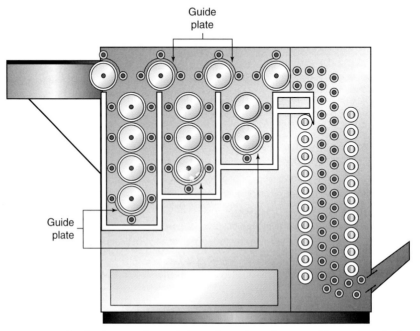

FIGURE 7-8 Guide plates are located throughout the roller assemblies and guide the leading edge of the moving film.

activates this motor. Most processors are also equipped with a standby control. The **standby control** is an electric circuit that shuts off power to the roller assemblies when the processor is not being used. Some wash water systems are also connected to the standby control. Pushing the standby control when ready to process a film can re-activate the roller assemblies and water intake. The standby control usually is on a timer so that several minutes after the last film has been processed, the standby circuit is activated and the rollers stop moving and wash water is no longer circulated. The purpose of this type of control is for cost-effectiveness. Decreasing motion of the rollers when processing is not occurring reduces the wear and tear on these assemblies. Water use can also decrease with use of a standby control. In addition, the standby control periodically reactivates the processor to keep chemicals mixed and temperatures stable throughout the tanks.

REPLENISHMENT SYSTEM

Replenishment refers to the replacement of fresh chemistry after the loss of chemistry during processing, specifically developer solution and fixer solution. The replenishment of chemicals used in the automatic processor is necessary because these chemicals eventually become exhausted and their ability to perform their functions decreases. Developer solution becomes exhausted through aerial oxidation and use oxidation.

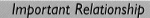

Important Relationship

Replenishment and Solution Performance

The replenishment system provides fresh chemistry to the developing and fixing solutions to maintain their chemical activity and volume when depleted during processing.

Aerial oxidation refers to a reduction in chemical strength as a result of exposure to air. **Use oxidation** refers to a reduction in chemical strength as a result of exposure to increased temperature over an extended period. Fixer solution becomes exhausted for several reasons: it becomes weakened simply from use, as a result of accumulations of silver halide that are removed from the film during the fixing process, and because of developer solution still present in the film, which decreases the strength and activity of the fixer solution. Two different types of replenishment systems are available. Many processors are equipped with the ability to use both types. One type of replenishment system bases the amount of solution to be replenished on the size of the film to be processed. This type of system uses microswitches that are connected to the entrance roller assembly (Figure 7-9). These microswitches are wired to two replenishment pumps, one for developer solution and one for fixer solution. As long as a piece of film is in the entrance roller assembly, the

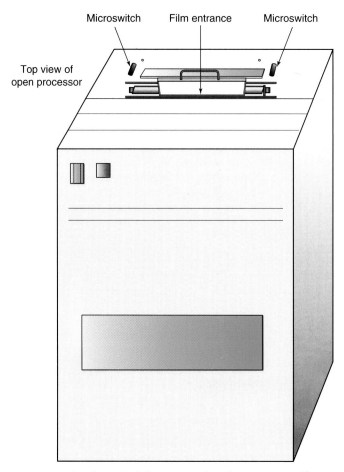

FIGURE 7-9 A microswitch is connected to the entrance roller assembly and activates the replenishment pumps while the film is in the entrance roller assembly.

microswitches and therefore the replenishment pumps will be activated. When the replenishment pumps are activated, they pump fresh solution from a reservoir system outside of the processor into the chemical tanks of the processor.

The volume of replenishment solution that is pumped into the chemical tanks is the same volume of used solution that is drained out of the processor. The amount of solution that is replenished is preset, although it can be adjusted, and depends on film size. For example, a film measuring 8×10 inches requires less volume of solutions than a film measuring 10×12 inches simply because of the difference in the physical area of both films. However, if an 8×10 inch film is run into the processor lengthwise and a 10×12 inch film is run in crosswise (Figure 7-10), the same volume of replenishment solutions will be pumped into the processor. This occurs

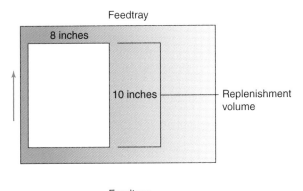

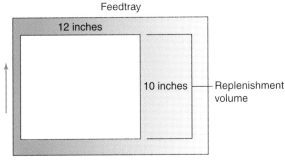

FIGURE 7-10 The volume of replenishment pumped into the processor is affected by the film dimension and its placement on the feedtray.

because the microswitch system hooked up to the entrance roller assembly senses the film while it is in the entrance roller assembly. The dimensions of the piece of film and how it is run into the processor determine the amount of time the replenishment pumps are activated. The running length of the film (Figure 7-11) determines how long the film will be in the entrance roller assembly and therefore the volume of replenishment solutions that will be pumped into the processor. It is important to run films into the processor in a particular orientation based on film size to avoid overreplenishment or underreplenishment of solutions.

Practical Tip

Film Orientation for Proper Replenishment

The radiographer should align the radiographic film so that the film is horizontally placed on the feedtray and its leading edge is long. When processing two 8 × 10 inch films, the radiographer should place both films parallel to each other so that the leading edges are short.

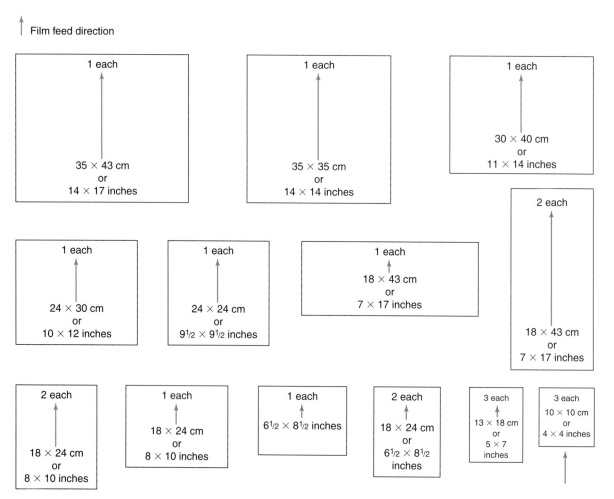

FIGURE 7-11 In general, radiographic film should be aligned so that the film is horizontally placed on the feedtray and its leading edge is long.

Overreplenishment of developer solution causes an increase in radiographic density and a decrease in radiographic contrast. Overreplenishment of fixer solution has no effect on radiographic quality but unnecessarily wastes solution. Underreplenishment of developer and fixer may cause films to jam in the roller transport system because of inadequate hardening of the film emulsion(s). Underreplenishment of developer can cause decreased density, whereas underreplenishment of fixer could result in poor archival quality of finished radiographs. Replenishment systems usually are adjusted so that more fixer solution is replenished per film in comparison to developer solution.

The second type of replenishment is called *flood replenishment.* **Flood replenishment** refers to the replenishment of solutions that occur at timed intervals, independent of the size or number of films processed. With flood replenishment, solutions

Developer orifice

Fixer orifice

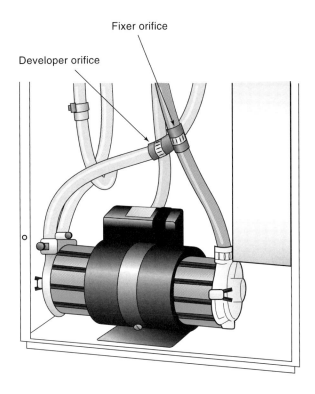

Figure 7-12 A recirculation system is located in the developer and fixer tanks to maintain solution activity and to provide the necessary agitation.

are pumped into the processor every several minutes while the motor drive of the processor is on standby. The timing of the intervals is adjustable. Flood replenishment is useful in processors that process a low to medium volume of films, especially single-emulsion films. In processors that are used in this manner, the stability of developer solution and radiographic density is difficult to maintain. Developer replenisher that contains starter solution is used in conjunction with flood replenishment to maintain developer solution activity and to produce more consistent levels of density on finished radiographs.

RECIRCULATION SYSTEM

Automatic processors have a recirculation system for the developer and fixer tanks. Each tank has a separate system that consists of a pump and connecting tubing. The **recirculation system** acts to circulate the solutions in each of these tanks by pumping solution out of one portion of the tank and returning it to a different location within the same tank from which it was removed (Figure 7-12). The recirculation system keeps the chemicals mixed, which helps maintain solution activity and provides agitation of the chemicals about the film to facilitate fast processing.

Important Relationship

Recirculation and Solution Performance

Recirculation of the developer and fixer solutions is necessary to maintain solution activity and the required agitation.

Recirculation also helps maintain the proper temperature of the developer solution. The developer recirculation system includes an in-line filter that removes impurities as the developer solution is being recirculated (Figure 7-13).

TEMPERATURE CONTROL

Temperature control of the developer solution is important because the activity of this solution heavily depends on its temperature. An increase or decrease in developer temperature can adversely affect the quality of the radiographic image.

Important Relationship

Developer Temperature and Radiographic Quality

Variations in developer temperature adversely affect the quality of the radiographic image. Increasing developer temperature increases the density, and decreasing developer temperature decreases the density. Radiographic contrast also may be adversely affected by changes in the developer temperature.

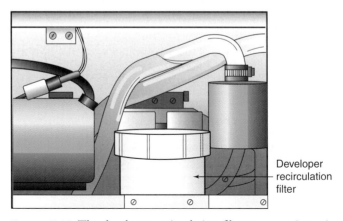

Developer recirculation filter

FIGURE 7-13 The developer recirculation filter removes impurities as the developer solution is being recirculated.

In most 90-second automatic processors, developer temperature must be maintained at 93° to 95° F (33.8° to 35° C). In older processors a mixing valve connected to the water input of the processor is used to mix hot and cold water to achieve the proper temperature of water entering the processor. This water is then circulated around the developer tank in water jackets to raise and maintain the temperature of the developer solution. In new processors an immersion heater (Figure 7-14) is used. An **immersion heater** is a heating coil that is immersed in the bottom of the developer tank. It is thermostatically controlled to heat the developer solution to its proper temperature and then maintain that temperature as long as the processor is turned on. Processors that use an immersion heater are sometimes called *cold-water processors* because they can adequately use a cold-water supply and do not depend on heated water for the heating of the developer solution. Developer temperature is usually displayed on the outside of the processor (Figure 7-15) as a convenience to the radiographer. Another possible way of controlling the temperature of the developer

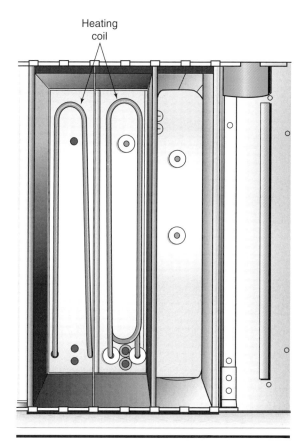

FIGURE 7-14 Top view of the inside of processor tanks. The immersion heater coil at the bottom of the developer tank heats and maintains the developer temperature.

solution is by using an in-line heat exchanger that is connected to the developer re-circulation system. As developer solution is recirculated, it passes through the thermostatically controlled heat exchanger and is heated to proper temperature.

DRYING SYSTEM

Radiographs must be properly dried to be viewed and stored. There are several means by which this may occur. The crossover roller assembly between the wash tank and the dryer contains several sets of squeegee rollers that remove some moisture from the film.

Important Relationship

Moisture and Archival Quality

The dryer assembly controls the amount of moisture removal to maintain the archival quality of radiographic film.

With large 90-second processors, as the film moves through the dryer, it is further dried by hot air that is blown onto both surfaces of the film. This air is forced through

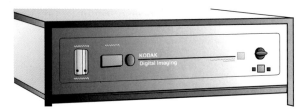

FIGURE 7-15 Developer temperature display.

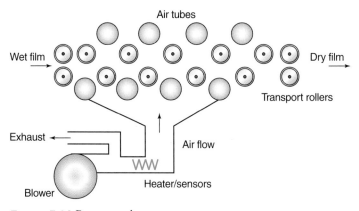

FIGURE 7-16 Processor dryer system.

the dryer by a blower and is directed onto the film by air tubes. The temperature of the air that is used to dry films is thermostatically monitored to accurately control moisture removal from the film (Figure 7-16). Some processors, especially slower and smaller tabletop models, may use infrared lamps instead of heated air to dry films.

Inadequate Processing

Inadequate processing is evidenced by certain appearances of the finished radiograph. Particular problems can be pinpointed by analyzing of the radiographs. These problems and the radiographic appearances that indicate them are summarized in Table 7-3.

TABLE 7-3   INDICATORS OF INADEQUATE PROCESSING

Radiographic Appearance	Processing Problem
Decrease in density	Developer exhausted Developer underreplenishment Processor running too fast Low developer temperature Developer improperly mixed
Increase in density	Developer overreplenishment High developer temperature Light leak in processor Developer improperly mixed
Pinkish stain (dichroic fog)	Contamination of developer by fixer Developer or fixer underreplenishment
Brown stain (thiosulfate stain)	Inadequate washing
Emulsion removed by developer	Insufficient hardener in developer
Milky appearance	Fixer exhausted Inadequate washing
Streaks	Dirty processor rollers Inadequate washing Inadequate drying
Water spots	Inadequate drying
Minus-density scratches	Scratches from guide plates caused by roller or plate misalignment

Film-Handling Areas

Film-handling areas in a radiology department include areas where unexposed film is stored, areas where radiographs are stored, and the processing area. Some important factors must be considered in these areas so that radiographic quality can be optimal.

STORING UNEXPOSED FILM

Unexposed film should be stored in its original packaging so that important information about the film can be maintained. Box 7-1 presents information that is contained on the outside of film boxes.

BOX 7-1 *Information Found on the Outside of Radiographic Film Boxes*

Brand name	Number of sheets
Expiration date	Safelight requirements
Lot number	Size
Manufacturer	

Film boxes should be stored vertically, not horizontally, to prevent pressure artifacts on the film. Film should be stored at a temperature ranging from 50° to 70° F (10° to 21° C) and a relative humidity of 40% to 60%. Film should be stored away from heat sources and ionizing radiation. Both heat and radiation can cause the silver halide in film emulsion to break down, causing the film to fog (Box 7-2). The shelf life of film, as expressed by its expiration date, must be observed. Film should not be used beyond this date. A FIFO system of rotation should be used to ensure that stored film is rotated properly into the film bin for immediate use. **FIFO** is an acronym for first in/first out, and this system requires that the film that is first received be the film that is first rotated out into the working film supply. This is contrasted with a LIFO (last in/first out) system that would ensure that only the freshest film is being used, while allowing older film to go to waste as it passes its expiration date.

BOX 7-2 *Possible Consequences of Storing Unexposed Film in Environments with Improper Temperature and Relative Humidity*

Storage Environment Problem	Possible Consequence
Temperature too high	Increased fog levels
Temperature too low	Increased static discharge
Humidity too high	Increased fog levels
Humidity too low	Increased static discharge

STORING RADIOGRAPHS

To ensure the stability of film emulsions, the radiographer should store finished radiographs within a range of particular temperatures and values of relative humidity. Specifically, radiographs should be stored between 60° and 80° F (16° to 26° C) and between 30% and 50% relative humidity. Also, although radiographic film generally has a "safety" designation that indicates it is nonflammable, the paper file folders that films are stored in are flammable. The area in which radiographs are stored should be designated as a no-smoking area, and the radiographs should be stored on metal shelving as opposed to wood shelving to further decrease the fire hazard.

The space needs for the storage of radiographs is considerable for many radiology departments. Stored radiographs can potentially take up a lot of valuable space within the department. Many departments use remote storage sites, either on site at their respective facilities or off site for the long-term storage of radiographs. The miniaturization of radiographs in the form of microfilm, microfiche, or 35-mm film has also become popular. Storing images digitally on computer disks or tape is becoming increasingly popular and will undoubtedly continue to rise in popularity.

The need for security of stored radiographs is also an important consideration. Radiographs are legally considered part of the patient's medical records, giving ownership of and responsibility for those records to the institution that produced them. Access to radiographs must be well controlled. Many facilities are finding it advantageous to not release original radiographs to requesting parties but instead to release duplicated copies of radiographs. This ensures that the patient's medical records are intact, despite the nonreturn of released radiographs to the lending facility.

THE DARKROOM

The darkroom in a radiology department is an obvious focal point of film handling. How film is handled in the darkroom can have a profound effect on the radiographs produced in a department. Common hazards to radiographic quality that can be found in the darkroom are white-light exposure, safelight exposure, ionizing radiation exposure, and other potential hazards.

Darkrooms must be free from all outside white-light exposure. A white-light source may be located inside the darkroom, but it should be connected to an interlock system whereby the film bin may not be opened as long as the darkroom light is on.

Safelights used in the darkroom must be equipped with a safelight filter that is appropriate for the type of film(s) being handled in the darkroom. Commonly used filters include Kodak Wratten 6B for blue-sensitive film and Kodak GBX for orthochromatic film, which is sensitive to both blue-violet and green visible light. Safelight filters must be free of cracks because otherwise white light from the safelight could leak in and expose the film. The power rating of the light bulbs used in safelights should be no greater than that which is recommended by film manufacturers (generally 7.5 to 15 W) and that which is indicated on the outside of the box of radiographic film.

Ionizing radiation exposure to film in the darkroom is a potential hazard because many darkrooms share common walls with radiographic rooms. The walls that are common with the darkroom and a radiographic room must be lined with lead as required by law for standard protection from radiographic exposures. The film bin where film is stored and available for immediate use should also be lead lined to prevent fog that may result from radiation exposure.

Other potential hazards to film in the darkroom include heat and chemical exposure. Film stored within the darkroom should not be close to any heat source. Processing chemicals must be kept away from film and film-handling areas to prevent exposure and contamination of these areas.

The darkroom should be centrally located to radiographic rooms for immediate access to these rooms. Although the radiologists' reading area may be some distance away, there should be some film-viewing capability close to the darkroom to allow radiographers the opportunity to assess their radiographs immediately after processing.

Darkrooms may be equipped with a single door, a revolving door, or a maze access. The color of interior walls should be light to reflect the small amount of light available from safelights. Floors should be of some material that makes them nonslippery when wet in the event of chemical or water spills or leaks inside the darkroom.

Unfortunately, darkrooms are not given much space within most radiology departments, so work space and storage space must be maximized. Countertops for film handling while loading and unloading cassettes must be free of excessive objects. Countertops must be clean and static free to avoid the formation of radiographic artifacts on the films. Several brands of commercial cleaning fluid that contain an antistatic component ideal for cleaning darkroom countertops and processor feedtrays are available. In addition, the floor space of the darkroom must be free of stored objects that one could trip over in the darkened environment.

Processing Quality Control

A quality control program must be implemented and systematically performed to ensure proper processing of radiographic film. A good quality control program will monitor all of the equipment and activities required for producing quality radiographic images. Radiographic quality cannot be achieved when film is improperly stored, mishandled before or after exposure, or incorrectly processed.

Silver Recovery

Because fixer solution is used to remove unexposed silver halide from the film, used fixer solution contains a high concentration of accumulated silver. Silver is considered a heavy metal, and disposing of it is regulated by local and state agencies. In many locales very strict limits are placed on the concentrations of silver in used fixer that can be disposed into the sewer system. Some type of silver recovery must be done when radiographic processing accumulates high concentrations of silver. **Silver recovery** refers to the removal of silver from used fixer solution. For some facilities regularly processing large volumes of radiographs, the financial rewards of silver recovery may be an added incentive.

The crudest and simplest method of silver recovery is to drain used fixer into a holding tank or container for retrieval by an appropriate silver recycler. This method is most appropriate for facilities that process a low volume of radiographs. The recycler must make regular visits to the facility or be called to retrieve the used fixer when the holding tank or container is full.

Silver-recovery units are available for on-site silver recovery and generally require servicing by an outside contractor who is familiar with the equipment and its method of removing silver. These silver-recovery units are connected directly to the drain system of the fixer tank to remove silver as used fixer solution passes through the unit. After the silver has been recovered, the used fixer then goes down the drain.

Silver-recovery units work by one of two methods. One method of silver recovery is called *metallic replacement.* Metallic replacement silver-recovery units can be of one of two types: one that uses steel wool and one that uses a silver-extraction filter. A steel wool metallic replacement unit uses steel wool to filter the used fixer solution. Silver replaces the iron in the steel wool and can then be removed easily after significant accumulation in a canister or replacement cartridge occurs. A silver-extraction–type unit uses a foam filter that is impregnated with steel wool. Again, the silver from used fixer solution replaces the iron in the steel wool. A silver-extraction filter is more efficient at removing silver from used fixer and lasts longer than a simple steel wool metallic replacement unit.

Another method of silver recovery is electrolytic. The electrolytic method is the most efficient method, but these units are also more expensive than metallic replacement units. Electrolytic units have an electrically charged drum or disk that attracts silver. The silver plates onto the drum or disk and can be removed when a substantial amount of silver has been collected.

Radiographic Artifacts

An **artifact** is any unwanted image on a radiograph. Artifacts are detrimental to radiographs because they can make visibility of anatomy, a pathologic condition, or patient identification information difficult or impossible. They decrease the overall radiographic quality of the image. Artifacts can be classified as *plus density* and *minus density.* Plus-density artifacts are greater in density than the area of the radiograph immediately surrounding them. Plus-density artifacts that are not caused by processing problems are presented in Table 7-4. Minus-density artifacts are of less density than the area of the radiograph immediately surrounding them. Some minus-density artifacts not caused by processing problems are presented in Table 7-5. For artifacts that result from processing problems, refer to Table 7-3.

TABLE 7-4   SOME COMMON PLUS-DENSITY ARTIFACTS NOT CAUSED BY PROCESSING

Artifact	Cause
Half-moon marks (Figure 7-17)	Bending or kinking of film before exposure
Scratches, abrasions (Figure 7-18)	Fingernail or other scratches before exposure

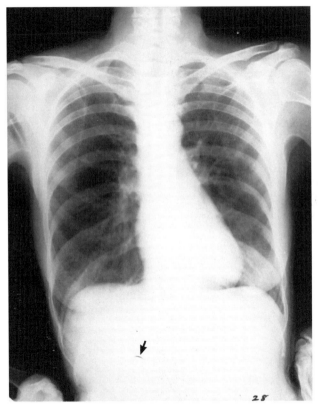
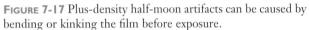
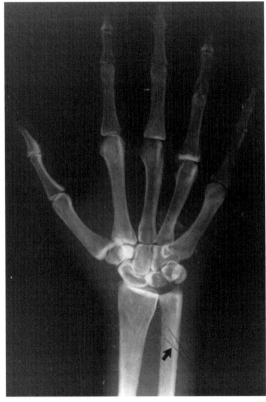

FIGURE 7-17 Plus-density half-moon artifacts can be caused by bending or kinking the film before exposure.

FIGURE 7-18 Plus-density scratch artifacts can be caused by a fingernail before exposure.

TABLE 7-4	SOME COMMON PLUS-DENSITY ARTIFACTS NOT CAUSED BY PROCESSING—cont'd
Artifact	**Cause**
Static discharges (Figure 7-19)	Sliding films over flat surface
Fogging	Exposure to white light, ionizing radiation, heat, safelight fogging; expired film
Density outside of collimated area	Off-focus or "off-stem" radiation

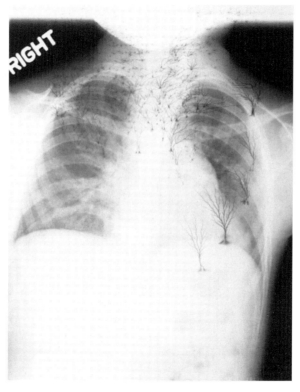

FIGURE 7-19 Plus-density static discharge artifact can be caused by sliding a film over a flat surface.

TABLE 7-5   SOME COMMON MINUS-DENSITY ARTIFACTS

Artifact	Cause
Fingerprints (Figure 7-20)	Moisture on finger transferred to film before exposure
Scratches, abrasions (Figure 7-21)	Fingernail or other scratches after exposure

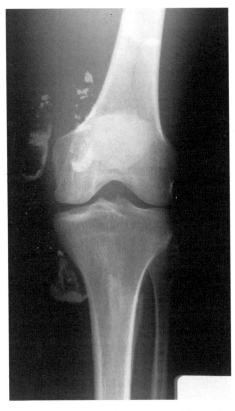

FIGURE 7-20 Minus-density caused by moisture on finger before exposure.

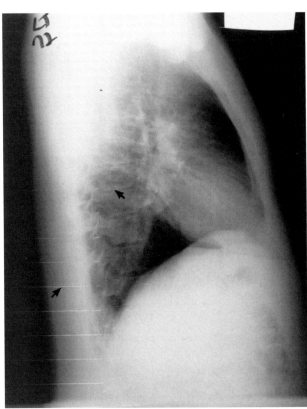

FIGURE 7-21 Minus-density scratch artifacts can be caused by transport rollers.

TABLE 7-5   SOME COMMON MINUS-DENSITY ARTIFACTS—cont'd

Artifact	Cause
Foreign object (Figure 7-22)	Some unintended object in the imaging chain
Nonspecific density decrease (Figure 7-23)	Dirty screens or cassette

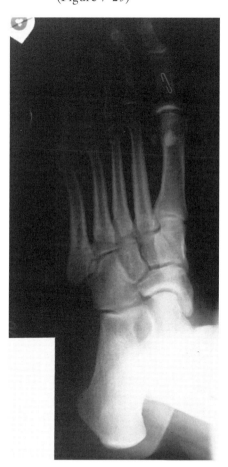

FIGURE 7-22 An unintended foreign object on the radiograph results in a minus-density artifact.

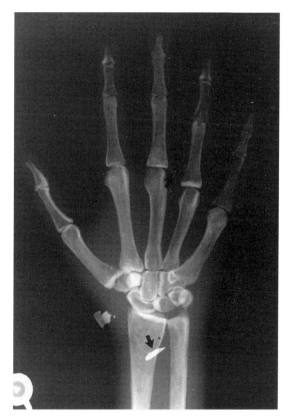

FIGURE 7-23 Dirty screens or cassettes can cause non-specific minus density artifacts.

Review Questions

1. Conversion of the latent to the manifest image is accomplished by
   A. the Gurney-Mott theory.
   B. radiographic processing.
   C. diffusion.
   D. oxidation.

2. The sequential order for processing radiographic film is
   A. developing, washing, fixing, drying.
   B. fixing, washing, developing, drying.
   C. developing, fixing, washing, drying.
   D. fixing, developing, washing, drying.

3. Which of the following solutions are responsible for reducing the exposed silver halide crystals to black metallic silver: 1.) ammonium thiosulfate, 2.) hydroquinone, or 3.) phenidone?
   A. 1 and 2 only
   B. 1 and 3 only
   C. 2 and 3 only
   D. 1, 2, and 3

4. The chemical responsible for maintaining the alkalinity of the developing solution is
   A. sodium carbonate.
   B. phenidone.
   C. acetic acid.
   D. sodium sulfite.

5. The fixing agent used to clear the undeveloped silver halide crystals is
   A. hydroquinone.
   B. aluminum chloride.
   C. potassium bromide.
   D. ammonium thiosulfate.

6. Staining or fading of the permanent image results when too much _____ remains on the film with improper washing.
   A. phenidone
   B. acetic acid
   C. thiosulfate
   D. glutaraldehyde

7. Finished radiographs should retain what percentage of their moisture?
   A. 2% to 5%
   B. 10% to 15%
   C. 20% to 30%
   D. 35% to 45%

8. The type of roller responsible for moving the film from the bottom of the tank upward is a(n) _____ roller.
   A. transport
   B. entrance
   C. turnaround
   D. crossover

9. The type of roller responsible for moving the film from one tank to another is a(n) _____ roller.
   A. transport
   B. entrance
   C. turnaround
   D. crossover

10. Processing chemicals must be replenished to maintain activity and volume when depleted primarily by
    A. oxidation.
    B. diffusion.
    C. precipitation.
    D. condensation.

11. Decreasing the developer temperature
    A. decreases oxidation.
    B. increases contrast.
    C. decreases density.
    D. increases processing time.

12. Under what environmental conditions should radiographic film be stored?
   A. Temperature between 40° and 60° F and 40% and 60% relative humidity
   B. Temperature between 50° and 70° F and 50% and 70% relative humidity
   C. Temperature between 40° and 60° F and 50% and 70% relative humidity
   D. Temperature between 50° and 70° F and 40% and 60% relative humidity

13. Safelight filters are chosen based on the
   A. amount of light intensity.
   B. dimensions of the darkroom.
   C. film sensitivity.
   D. power rating.

14. The type of silver-recovery unit that uses an electrically charged drum to attract the silver is called a(n) _____ unit.
   A. an extraction filter
   B. electrolytic
   C. steel wool
   D. metallic replacement

15. A common plus-density artifact caused from bending the film before exposure is
   A. half-moon marks.
   B. static discharge.
   C. abrasion.
   D. fogging.

CHAPTER 8

Sensitometry

USE OF SENSITOMETRY

EQUIPMENT

Penetrometer
Sensitometer
Densitometer

OPTICAL DENSITY

Diagnostic Range

SENSITOMETRIC CURVE

Log of Relative Exposure
Regions

FILM CHARACTERISTICS

Speed
Contrast
Exposure Latitude

CLINICAL CONSIDERATIONS

Optimal Density
Maximum Film Contrast

REVIEW QUESTIONS

1 Define all of the key terms in this chapter.

2 State all of the important relationships in this chapter.

3 Explain the importance of sensitometry to radiography.

4 Define *optical density* and explain its logarithmic scale.

5 State the diagnostic range of optical densities.

6 Given an optical density, convert it to its percentage of light transmission.

7 Explain the construction of sensitometric curves.

8 Identify all regions of a sensitometric curve.

9 Describe the characteristics of sensitometric curves.

10 Differentiate among the film characteristics of speed, contrast, and latitude.

11 Given sensitometric curves, compare their characteristics.

12 Calculate film speed and average gradient.

13 Evaluate the effect of exposure technique on the film characteristics of density and contrast.

KEY TERMS

sensitometry
intensity of radiation exposure
penetrometer
step-wedge densities
sensitometer
sensitometer strip
densitometer
optical density (OD)
logarithmic scale
base plus fog (B + F)
sensitometric curve
log relative exposure
toe region
D_{min}
straight-line region

shoulder region
D_{max}
speed
speed point
speed exposure point
antilog
film contrast
slope
gradient point
average gradient
gamma
exposure latitude
optimal density
maximum contrast

In radiography, **sensitometry** is the study of the relationship between the intensity of radiation exposure to the film and the amount of blackness produced after processing (density). The **intensity of radiation exposure** is the measurement of the quantity of radiation reaching an area of the film.

Use of Sensitometry

Sensitometry provides a method of evaluating the characteristics of film and film-screen combinations used in radiography. Radiographic film and intensifying screen manufacturers are capable of designing film and screens to respond differently to a given intensity of radiation exposure. Film and screens designed for radiography of the chest or extremities respond differently to equal amounts of radiation exposure. It is important for the radiographer to understand how the film and film-screen system used will respond to a given intensity of exposure.

Sensitometry is also a method of evaluating the performance of automatic processors. Because automatic processors affect a radiograph's density and contrast, the variability of its performance can be monitored by sensitometric methods.

Equipment

Several pieces of equipment are needed to evaluate the relationship between the intensity of radiation exposure and the density produced after processing. The radiographic film needs to be exposed to a range of radiation intensities to evaluate its response to low, middle, and high exposures. This can be accomplished easily by using a radiographic x-ray unit and passing the radiation through an object that varies in thickness. The resultant effect is an image of varying uniform densities that correspond to a specific intensity of radiation exposure.

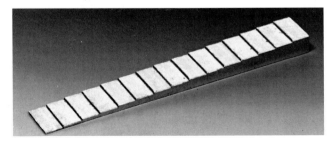

FIGURE 8-1 A penetrometer. When radiographed, a penetrometer produces an image showing a series of uniform densities.

PENETROMETER

A **penetrometer** is a device constructed of uniform absorbers of increasing thicknesses, such as aluminum or tissue-equivalent plastic (Figure 8-1). When radiographed, the penetrometer produces a series of uniform densities that resemble a step wedge (Figure 8-2). When **step-wedge densities** are produced with a penetrometer and a radiographic x-ray unit, the variability of the output of the equipment could affect the range of densities produced.

SENSITOMETER

A device known as a **sensitometer** is designed to produce consistent step-wedge densities by eliminating the variability of the x-ray unit (Figure 8-3). It uses a controlled light source to expose an optical step-wedge template. The step-wedge template transmits light in varying intensities to expose the radiographic film. After the film has been processed, a density step-wedge image, or **sensitometric strip,** is produced. Penetrometers and sensitometers are available in 11-, 15-, or 21-step densities.

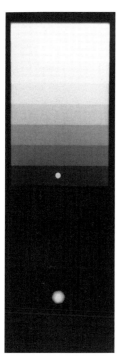

FIGURE 8-2 Radiograph of a penetrometer showing step-wedge densities.

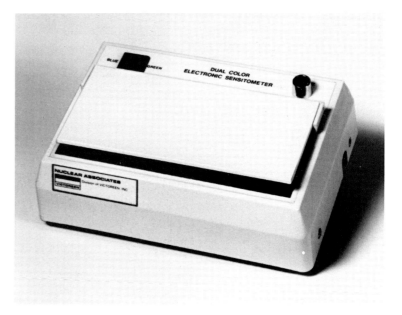

FIGURE 8-3 A sensitometer is designed to produce consistent step-wedge densities. *Courtesy Nuclear Associates.*

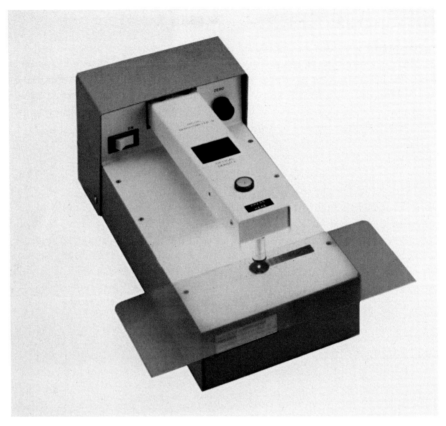

FIGURE 8-4 A densitometer is used to measure optical densities. *Courtesy Nuclear Associates.*

DENSITOMETER

A **densitometer** is a device used to numerically determine the amount of blackness on the film after processing (i.e., it measures radiographic density). This device is constructed to emit a constant intensity of light (incident) onto an area of film and then measure the amount of light transmitted through the film (Figure 8-4). The densitometer determines the amount of light transmitted and calculates a measurement known as **optical density (OD).**

Optical Density

Optical density is a numeric calculation that compares the amount of light transmitted through an area of radiographic film to the amount of light originally striking (incident) the film. Box 8-1 shows the mathematical formula used.

Box 8-1 *Light Transmittance Formula*

$$\frac{I_t}{I_o} \times 100$$

where I_t represents the amount of light transmitted and I_o represents the amount of original light incident on the film.

Because the range of radiographic densities is large, the calculation of radiographic densities is compressed into a **logarithmic scale** (Table 8-1) for easier management.

A film that allows 100% of the original incident light to be transmitted through will have a logarithmic value of 0. A film that allows only 1% of the original incident

TABLE 8-1	PERCENTAGE OF LIGHT TRANSMITTANCE AND CALCULATED OPTICAL DENSITIES	
Percentage of Light Transmitted ($I_t/I_o \times 100$)	**Fraction of Light Transmitted (I_t/I_o)**	**Optical Density (log I_o/I_t)**
100	1	0
50	1/2	0.3
32	8/25	0.5
25	1/4	0.6
12.5	1/8	0.9
10	1/10	1
5	1/20	1.3
3.2	4/125	1.5
2.5	1/30	1.6
1.25	1/80	1.9
1	1/100	2
0.5	1/200	2.3
0.32	2/625	2.5
0.125	1/800	2.9
0.1	1/1000	3
0.05	1/2000	3.3
0.032	1/3125	3.5
0.01	1/10,000	4

light through will have a logarithmic value of 2.0. This logarithmic value of light transmittance is termed *optical density*. The formula used to calculate optical density is shown in Box 8-2.

BOX 8-2 *Optical Density Formula*

$$\text{Optical density} = \text{Log}_{10} \frac{I_o}{I_t}$$

where I_o represents the amount of original light incident on the film and I_t represents the amount of transmitted light.

Important Relationship

Light Transmittance and Optical Density

As the percentage of light transmitted decreases, the optical density increases; as the percentage of light transmitted increases, the optical density decreases.

Notice the relationship between light transmittance and optical density. When 100% of the light is transmitted, the optical density equals 0.0. When 50% of the light is transmitted, the optical density is equal to 0.3, and when 25% of the light is transmitted, the optical density equals 0.6. When a logarithmic scale base 10 is used, every 0.3 change in optical density corresponds to a change in the percentage of light transmitted by a factor of 2 ($\log_{10}$ of $2 = 0.3$).

Important Relationship

Optical Density and Light Transmittance

For every 0.3 change in optical density, the percentage of light transmitted has changed by a factor of 2. A 0.3 increase in optical density results from a decrease in the percentage of light transmitted by half, whereas a 0.3 decrease in optical density results from an increase in the percentage of light transmitted by a factor of 2.

Optical densities can range from 0.0 to 4.0 OD. Because most radiographic film has a tint added to its base and processing adds a slight amount of fog, the lowest amount of optical density is usually between 0.10 and 0.20 OD. This minimum amount of density on the radiographic film is termed the **base plus fog (B + F).**

DIAGNOSTIC RANGE

In radiography the useful range of optical densities is between 0.25 and 2.5 OD. However, the diagnostic range of optical densities for general radiography usually falls between 0.5 and 2.0 OD. This desired range of optical densities is found between the extreme low and high densities produced on the film.

Sensitometric Curve

When the optical density measurements from a sensitometric strip are graphed, the result is a curve characteristic of the radiographic film type. Box 8-3 lists other terms used for the **sensitometric curve.**

Box 8-3   *Other Terms for Sensitometric Curve*

Characteristic curve
D log E curve
H & D curve
Hurter & Driffield curve

This sensitometric curve visually demonstrates the relationship between the intensity of radiation exposure (x axis) and the resultant optical densities (y axis) (Figure 8-5). The position of the curve on the x axis and its shape can vary greatly depending on the type of radiographic film used.

LOG OF RELATIVE EXPOSURE

When sensitometric methods are used to evaluate the characteristics of radiographic film, it is more useful to measure the intensity of radiation exposure in increments of a constant change, such as doubling or halving. Remember that for every doubling or halving change in the percentage of light transmitted, a 0.3 change in optical density occurs. Along the x axis, for every 0.3 change in **log relative exposure,** the intensity of radiation exposure changes by a factor of 2 (Figure 8-6). Using Figure 8-6, notice for the log exposure of 1.5, the relative mAs (the product of milliamperage and exposure time) value is 32, and for the log of exposure 1.8, the relative mAs value is 64. This relationship can be demonstrated throughout the log relative exposure scale on the sensitometric curve. Two exposures, one double the other, will always be separated by 0.3 on the logarithmic exposure scale.

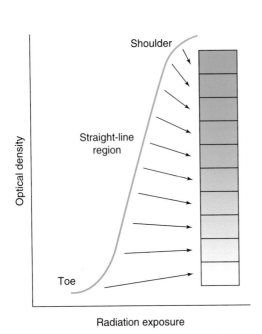

FIGURE 8-5 Plotting optical densities corresponding to the change in intensity of exposure results in a curve characteristic of the type of the film.

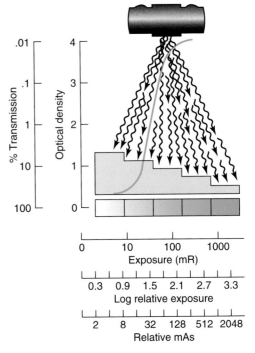

FIGURE 8-6 A sensitometric curve is created by plotting the optical density values obtained from the range of exposures that are used to create the step-wedge densities. The log relative exposure value representing the change in exposure by a factor of 2 is a more useful value than the milliroentgen (mR) exposure or relative mAs.

Important Relationship

Log Relative Exposure

A 0.3 change in log of exposure represents a change in intensity of radiation exposure by a factor of 2. An increase of 0.3 log of exposure results in a doubling of the amount of radiation exposure, whereas a decrease in 0.3 log of exposure results in halving the amount of radiation exposure.

REGIONS

A sensitometric curve demonstrates three distinct regions (Figure 8-7). When the characteristics of different types of radiographic film are evaluated, differences will be demonstrated within any of these regions.

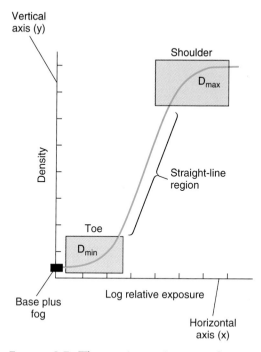

FIGURE 8-7 The sensitometric curve demonstrates three distinct regions: toe, straight-line, and shoulder.

Toe Region

The **toe region** of the sensitometric curve represents the area of low density. The point on the sensitometric curve where the minimum amount of radiation exposure produced a minimum amount of optical density is known as D_{min}. Generally, the D_{min} will be equal to B + F even though they represent two different measurements. Changes in exposure intensity in this region have little effect on the optical density.

Straight-Line Region

At some point along the x axis, changes in exposure begin to have a much greater effect on the optical density. This **straight-line region** is where the diagnostic or most useful range of densities is produced.

Shoulder Region

There is a point on the sensitometric curve where changes in exposure intensity no longer greatly affect the optical density. In this **shoulder region,** the point on the curve where maximum density has been produced is known as D_{max}. Once the maximum density achievable within the film has been reached (D_{max}), continued increases in exposure intensity will begin to reverse the amount of optical density. This process is called *solarization*, and it is the process used in the design of duplicating film.

Film Characteristics

Comparing sensitometric curves on these regions provides information about three important characteristics of the radiographic film. Each film characteristic plays an important role in radiographic imaging.

SPEED

An important characteristic of radiographic film is its sensitivity to radiation exposure, referred to as its **speed.** The speed of a film indicates the amount of optical density produced for a given amount of radiation exposure. It is a characteristic of the film's sensitivity to the intensity of radiation exposure.

Important Relationship

Film Speed and Optical Density

For a given exposure, as the speed of a film increases, the optical density produced also increases; as the speed of a film decreases, the optical density decreases.

Speed Point

The speed of radiographic film typically is determined by locating the point on a sensitometric curve that corresponds to the optical density of 1.0 plus B + F. This point is called the **speed point** (Figure 8-8). This optical density point is used because it is within the straight-line portion of the sensitometric curve. The speed point serves as a standard method of indicating film speed.

Speed Exposure Point

When comparing film types, the radiographer must determine what log of exposure produced the speed point. This can be determined by drawing a line from the sensitometric curve speed point to the area on the x axis (log of exposure) that produced the optical density at 1.0 plus B + F (Figure 8-9). This important point, called the **speed exposure point,** indicates the intensity of exposure needed to

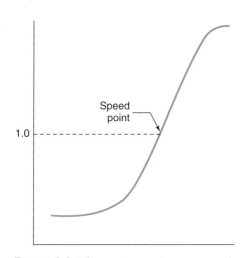

FIGURE 8-8 The sensitometric curve speed point indicates the intensity of exposure needed to produce a density of 1.0 plus base plus fog (speed point).

FIGURE 8-9 The speed exposure point indicates the intensity of exposure needed to produce a density of 1.0 plus base plus fog (speed point).

produce a density of 1.0 plus B + F (speed point). A film that has a speed exposure point of 0.9 is faster than a film having a speed exposure point of 1.2.

Important Relationship

Film Speed and Speed Exposure Point

The lower the speed exposure point, the faster the film speed; the higher the speed exposure point, the slower the film speed.

Figure 8-10 presents two sensitometric curves and their respective speed point and speed exposure point. Visually, it is apparent that a faster-speed film is positioned to the left (closer to the y axis) of slower-speed film.

Practical Tip

Sensitometric Curves Position along the X Axis

Sensitometric curves of faster-speed film are positioned to the left of slower-speed film, and sensitometric curves of slower-speed film are positioned to the right of faster-speed film.

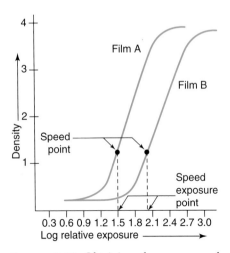

FIGURE 8-10 Obtaining the same speed point requires that Film A have a 1.5 log of exposure and Film B have a 2.0 log of exposure. Faster-speed films are located to the left of slower-speed films.

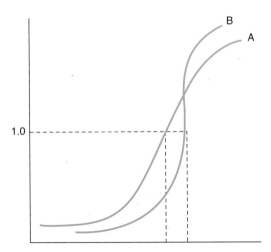

FIGURE 8-11 As the shape of the sensitometric curve varies, the speed can also vary if it is measured at points other than the standard of 1.0 plus base plus fog.

It is important to remember that the speed of the film is determined by the amount of exposure (log of exposure) needed to produce an optical density of 1.0 plus B + F, regardless of the shape of the sensitometric curve (Figure 8-11).

Film Speed Formula

The radiographer needs to comprehend the method used to compare various film speeds and their subsequent effect on exposure techniques. The film speed formula provides a mathematical calculation for the differences in film speed (Box 8-4).

BOX 8-4 *Film Speed Formula*

$$\text{Antilog } (E_2 - E_1)$$

Film A	**Film B**
$E_2 = 1.2$	$E_1 = 0.85$

$$\text{Antilog } (1.2 - 0.85)$$

Antilog $(0.35) = 2.24$. Film B is 2.24 times faster than Film A. This factorial change in intensity can then be applied to the actual mAs value to adjust the optical density accordingly.

Comparison of speed among different types of film will assist the radiographer in determining the changes needed in exposure technique to maintain comparable radiographic density. Calculating the **antilog** of the differences between two speed exposure points will demonstrate the factorial change in intensity of exposure. For example, the antilog of the exposure between Film A and Film B equals 2.24 (see Box 8-4). This represents a change in log of exposure by a factor of 2.24, or 224%. This means that Film B is 2.24 times faster than Film A. To maintain density when changing from Film B to Film A, the radiographer must increase the exposure technique by a factor of 2.24 (Film B mAs [20] × 2.24 = 44.8 new mAs for Film A).

This formula also can be used to calculate changes in exposure to alter the optical density for a given radiographic image: calculate the difference between the exposure points for the initial optical density point and the desired optical density point and find the antilog. As in the previous example with two different types of film, the antilog can be used to adjust the actual mAs to increase or decrease the optical densities on a repeated radiographic study.

X Mathematical Application

Using Sensitometry to Calculate Exposure Technique Changes

60 mAs produced an image density of 2.05 (log E = 1.54). What mAs would produce an image density of 1.30 (log E = 1.38)?

Subtract log E of the original density (2.05) from the log E of the desired density (1.30):

$$\begin{array}{r} 1.38 \\ -1.54 \\ \hline -0.16; \text{ antilog of } -0.16 = 0.69 \end{array}$$

Multiply the original mAs by 0.69:

$$60 \text{ mAs} \times 0.69 = 41.4 \text{ mAs}$$

Changing the original optical density on the repeat radiograph from 2.05 to 1.30 requires that the mAs needs be decreased to 41.4.

CONTRAST

Radiographic contrast is a result of both the subject contrast and the **film contrast.** Film contrast is controlled by the design and manufacturing of the film components and the effect of processing. The ability of a radiographic film to provide a level of contrast can be evaluated by the steepness, or **slope,** of the sensitometric curve. The slope of this line mathematically indicates the ratio of the change in y (optical density) for a unit change in x (log relative exposure) (Box 8-5).

BOX 8-5   *Determining the Slope of a Line*

$$\text{Slope} = \frac{Y \text{ (rise)}}{X \text{ (run)}}, \qquad \frac{y_2 - y_1}{x_2 - x_1}$$

The slope of a line mathematically indicates its tilt or slant. Comparisons of the slope (mathematical calculation) can be made among different lines. For radiography, the higher the number, the steeper the slope, and the lower the number, the lesser the slope.

Visually comparing the steepness (slope) of the straight-line region of the curve provides a method of evaluating the level of contrast produced by a film (Figure 8-12). Radiographic film capable of producing higher contrast will have a more vertical straight-line region (steeper slope).

Important Relationship

Slope and Film Contrast

The steeper the slope of the straight-line region (more vertical), the higher the film contrast; the lesser the slope (less vertical), the lower the film contrast.

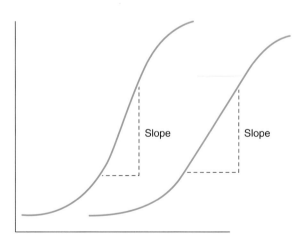

FIGURE 8-12 The slope of the straight-line region determines the inherent film contrast. Steeper slopes indicate higher contrast.

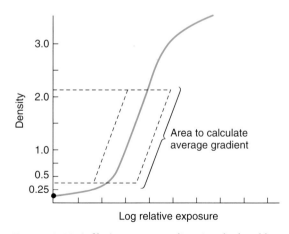

FIGURE 8-13 A film's average gradient is calculated between a low density (0.25 plus base plus fog) and a high density (2.0 plus base plus fog).

General-purpose radiographic film generally is categorized as either high contrast or medium contrast.

Gradient Point

Determining the slope along any portion of the sensitometric curve provides information about the contrast produced at that point, called the **gradient point.** Gradient points can be determined for any regions of the sensitometric curve, such as the toe, middle, and shoulder. The gradient point can be determined by calculating the slope of the line (change in optical density divided by the change in log exposure) at any portion of the curve.

Average Gradient

When evaluating film for comparison, the radiographer typically determines contrast by calculating the sensitometric curve's **average gradient** of the slope of the straight-line region (Figure 8-13). A standard used in sensitometry is to determine the contrast between the optical densities of 0.25 and 2.0 plus B + F. Finding the difference between these two points and dividing by the difference between their respective log of exposures provides a numerical calculation for film contrast. Most radiographic film will have an average gradient between 2.5 and 3.5.

 X   Mathematical Application

Calculating Average Gradient

$$\text{Average gradient} = \frac{D_2 - D_1}{E_2 - E_1}$$

where

$$D_1 = OD\ 0.25 + 0.17\ (B + F)$$
$$D_2 = OD\ 2.0 + 0.17\ (B + F)$$
$$E_1 = \text{Exposure that produces } D_1$$
$$E_2 = \text{Exposure that produces } D_2$$

Example:

$$\frac{2.17 - 0.42}{1.46 - 0.8} = \frac{1.75}{0.66} = 2.65 \text{ Average gradient}$$

Film contrast will be higher for a film with an average gradient of 3.0 compared with that of a film having an average gradient of 2.7.

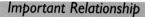

Important Relationship

Average Gradient and Film Contrast

The greater the average gradient, the higher the film contrast; the lower the average gradient, the lower the film contrast.

Gamma

Gamma is another gradient point that is calculated from points surrounding the optical density of 1.0 found within the straight-line region of the sensitometric curve.

Gradient point, average gradient, and gamma all provide information about the contrast produced by a type of radiographic film. To make equal comparisons of the characteristics of film, the radiographer must determine the contrast by using the same method.

EXPOSURE LATITUDE

Exposure latitude refers to the range of exposures that will produce optical densities within the straight-line region of the sensitometric curve (Figure 8-14). Radiographic films that are capable of responding to a wide range of exposures to produce

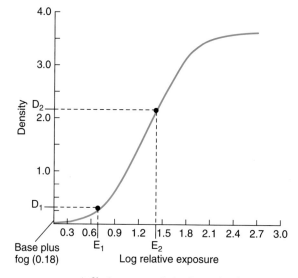

FIGURE 8-14 A film's exposure latitude can be determined by finding the range of exposures that will produce densities within the straight-line region of the curve. Using a low and high density similar to those used to calculate average gradient would provide optical densities within the straight-line region of the sensitometric curve.

optical densities within the straight-line region are considered wide-latitude film. When films are being compared, one with narrow latitude and one with wide latitude, it is visually apparent that a film with narrow latitude is a higher-contrast film and a film with wide latitude is a lower-contrast film (Figure 8-15). A steep slope has a small range of exposures available to produce densities within the straight-line region, whereas a less steep slope has a greater range of densities available to produce densities within the straight-line region.

Important Relationship

Exposure Latitude and Film Contrast

Exposure latitude and film contrast have an inverse relationship. High-contrast radiographic film will have narrow latitude, and low-contrast film will have wide latitude.

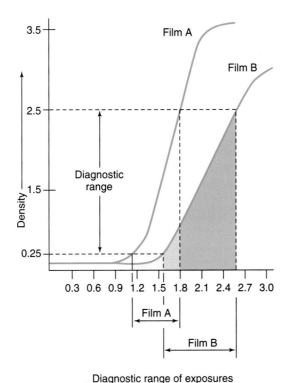

FIGURE 8-15 A higher-contrast film, Film A, has a narrower range of exposures available to produce optical densities within the straight-line region compared with a lower-contrast film, Film B.

When selecting a type of radiographic film to use, the radiographer should evaluate its characteristics in terms of speed, contrast, and latitude. Radiographic film used in chest radiography typically requires lower contrast and wider-exposure latitude, whereas film designed for use with skull radiography requires higher contrast, resulting in narrow-exposure latitude. The speed of radiographic film is considered in combination with the intensifying screen speed to provide a film-screen system speed.

Clinical Considerations

To provide radiographic images of optimal radiographic quality, the radiographer must control visibility factors of density and contrast appropriately. A relationship exists between density and contrast to maximize the amount of recorded detail visible.

OPTIMAL DENSITY

For a given anatomic area to be radiographed, exposure techniques selected should produce radiographic densities that will lie within the straight-line region of the sensitometric curve. Optical densities within this range will maximize the amount of information visible within the radiographic image, resulting in **optimal density.**

The challenge for radiographers is to determine the amount of radiation exposure necessary to produce optical densities within the straight-line region of a film's sensitometric curve. Different types of radiographic film may require different amounts of exposure to produce optical densities within the straight-line region. As demonstrated previously, it may take more or less radiation exposure to produce an optical density of 1.0 plus B + F for Film A as compared with Film B. Therefore the relationship between radiation exposure and optical density depends on the shape and position of a film's sensitometric curve.

For a given type of radiographic film, when optical densities lie within the straight-line region of the sensitometric curve, a change in exposure technique will have a direct change in optical density (Figure 8-16). When optical densities lie outside the range of the straight-line region, a greater or lesser change in exposure technique may be needed to move the optical densities back within the diagnostic range (0.5 to 2.0 OD). When evaluating a radiograph with a density error, the radiographer must determine the amount of change needed in the exposure technique to place the optical densities within the diagnostic range.

Practical Tip

Changes in Exposure Technique to Correct for Density Errors

Optical densities that lie outside the straight-line region of the sensitometric curve (toe or shoulder region) require a greater or lesser change in exposure than those that lie within the straight-line region to correct for the density error.

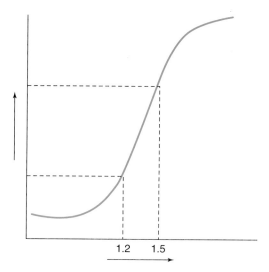

FIGURE 8-16 When optical densities lie within the straight-line region of the curve, a 0.3 change in log exposure (change by a factor of 2) produces a direct change in optical densities.

In diagnostic radiology one type of film generally is used for most procedures. Access to a film's sensitometric curve for the purpose of calculating exposure changes is not practical. Therefore it is the radiographer's responsibility to use the standard guidelines (discussed in Chapter 4) regarding exposure changes to correct for density errors.

MAXIMUM FILM CONTRAST

Film contrast is the difference in optical density between two points anywhere along the sensitometric curve (Figure 8-17). If these differences in optical density were plotted as points between the x and y axes, the result would be a film's contrast curve (Figure 8-18). When the contrast curve is evaluated, it is apparent that **maximum contrast** (the greatest difference in optical densities) is achievable within the straight-line region of the sensitometric curve. When optical densities of the anatomic area of interest lie outside the straight-line region, film contrast is decreased.

Practical Tip

Achieving Maximum Film Contrast

To achieve the maximum contrast that the film is capable of producing, the radiographer must ensure that the optical densities lie within the straight-line region of the sensitometric curve.

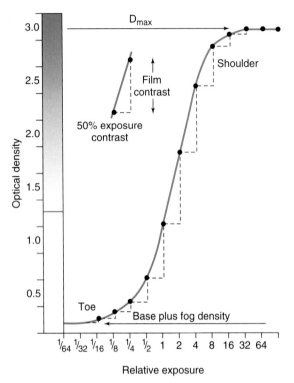

FIGURE 8-17 Density differences calculated along the sensitometric curve can be used to evaluate film contrast.

FIGURE 8-18 Plotting the density differences of a sensitometric curve results in a contrast curve. Maximum film contrast is achieved within the straight-line region.

When optical densities lie within the straight-line region of the sensitometric curve, the film has reached its maximum capability in visualizing recorded detail.

In summary, sufficient radiographic density is needed to visualize recorded detail. A film's maximum radiographic contrast can be visualized only when optical densities lie within the straight-line region of the sensitometric curve. When optical densities lie outside the straight-line region, film contrast is decreased. When both optimum density and maximum contrast have been achieved, the visibility of recorded details is of optimal radiographic quality.

Review Questions

1. What term is defined as *a measurement of the amount of light transmitted through the film?*
   A. Sensitometry
   B. Film contrast
   C. Film speed
   D. Optical density

2. What is the diagnostic range of optical densities?
   A. 0.15 to 4.0
   B. 0.25 to 2.0
   C. 0.5 to 1.25
   D. 0.10 to 2.0

3. An optical density of 1.0 indicates that _____ light was transmitted.
   A. 0.01%
   B. 0.1%
   C. 1.0%
   D. 10%

4. A _____ change in optical density results from a change in the percentage of light transmittance by a factor of 2.
   A. 0.03
   B. 0.3
   C. 3.0
   D. 30

5. Changes in exposure have little effect on density in which of the following regions of the sensitometric curve: 1.) toe, 2.) shoulder, or 3.) straight line?
   A. 1 and 2 only
   B. 1 and 3 only
   C. 2 and 3 only
   D. 1, 2, and 3

6. When the exposure technique used produces densities outside the straight-line portion of a sensitometric curve, how is contrast affected?
   A. Increased
   B. No effect
   C. Decreased
   D. Improved

7. Compare the sensitometric curves in Figure 8-19. Which film is faster?
   A. Film A
   B. Film B
   C. Film C
   D. Film D

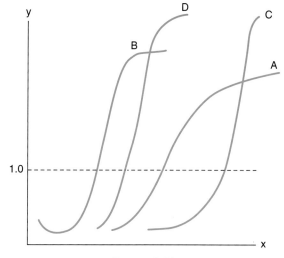

FIGURE 8-19

8. Compare the sensitometric curves in Figure 8-19. Which film has lower contrast?
   A. Film A
   B. Film B
   C. Film C
   D. Film D

9. Film B has an exposure speed point of 1.5, and Film A has an exposure speed point of 1.2. Is there a difference in speed?
   A. Film A is twice as fast as Film B.
   B. Film A and B have equal speed.
   C. Film A is half as fast as Film B.
   D. Film B is twice as fast as Film A.

10. Changes in radiation exposure minimally change optical densities in which sensitometric region?
   A. Toe
   B. Shoulder
   C. Straight-line
   D. A and B

CHAPTER 9

Exposure Factor Selection

EXPOSURE TECHNIQUE CHARTS

Conditions

Design Characteristics

TYPES OF TECHNIQUE CHARTS

Variable kVp/Fixed mAs
Technique Chart

Fixed kVp/Variable mAs
Technique Chart

**EXPOSURE TECHNIQUE
CHART DEVELOPMENT**

Development Stages

REVIEW QUESTIONS

The radiographer has the primary task of selecting the exposure factors that will produce a quality radiographic image. Many variables can affect the production of a quality radiograph. Previous chapters have discussed the exposure factors and their effect on the radiographic image. Knowledge of these factors and the qualities inherent in an optimal radiographic image will aid the radiographer in the selection of exposure factors for a particular radiographic examination. Exposure technique charts are useful tools to assist the radiographer in selecting a manual exposure technique or when using automatic exposure control (AEC). This chapter focuses on the design and use of exposure technique charts to assist the radiographer in the consistent production of quality radiographic images.

Exposure Technique Charts

Exposure technique charts are preestablished guidelines used by the radiographer to select standardized manual or AEC exposure factors for each type of radiographic examination. Technique charts standardize the selection of exposure factors for the typical patient so that the quality of radiographic images is consistent.

For each radiographic procedure, the radiographer consults the technique chart for the recommended exposure variables—kilovoltage peak (kVp), mAs (the product of milliamperage and exposure time), film-screen combination, grid, and source-to-image receptor distance (SID). Based on the thickness of the anatomic part to be radiographed, the radiographer selects the exposure factors presented in the technique chart. For example, a patient is scheduled for a routine abdominal examination. The radiographer positions the patient and aligns the central ray (CR) to the patient and image receptor, measures the abdomen for a manual technique, and consults the chart for the predetermined standardized exposure variables.

Because many factors have an impact on the selection of appropriate exposure factors, technique charts are instrumental in the production of consistent quality radiographs, reduction in repeat radiographic studies, and reduction in patient exposure. The proper development and use of technique charts are keys to the selection of appropriate exposure factors.

Important Relationship

Exposure Technique Charts and Radiographic Quality

A properly designed and used technique chart standardizes the selection of exposure factors to help the radiographer produce consistent quality radiographs while minimizing patient exposure.

CONDITIONS

A technique chart presents exposure factors that are to be used for a particular examination given the type of radiographic equipment. Technique charts help ensure that consistent image quality is achieved throughout the entire radiology department; they also decrease the number of repeat radiographic studies needed and therefore decrease the patient's exposure.

Technique charts will not replace the critical thinking skills required of the radiographer. The radiographer must continue to use individual judgment and discretion in properly selecting exposure factors for each patient and type of examination. The radiographer's primary task is to produce the highest quality radiograph while delivering the least amount of radiation exposure. Technique charts are designed for the average or typical patient and do not account for unusual circumstances. These atypical conditions require accurate patient assessment and appropriate exposure technique adjustment by the radiographer. See Chapter 11 for details regarding these situations.

 Practical Tip

Technique Chart Limitations

Exposure technique charts are designed for the typical or average patient. Patient variability in terms of body habitus, physical condition, or the presence of a pathologic condition requires the radiographer to problem solve when selecting exposure factors.

A technique chart needs to be established for each x-ray tube, even if a single generator is used for more than one tube. For example, if a radiographic room has two x-ray tubes, one for a radiographic table and one for an upright Bucky unit, each tube needs to have its own technique chart because of possible inherent differences in the exposure output produced by each tube. Each portable radiographic unit must also have its own technique chart.

For technique charts to be effective tools in producing consistent quality radiographs, departmental standards for radiographic quality need to be determined. In addition, standardization of exposure factors and the use of accessory devices are needed. For example, the adult knee can be radiographed adequately with or without the use of a grid. Although both radiographs might be acceptable, departmental standards may prefer the radiograph to be imaged with the use of a grid. These types of decisions need to be made before technique chart development takes place so that the departmental standards can be clarified. Technique charts are then constructed using these standards, and radiographers should adhere to the departmental standards.

Two conditions absolutely must be met for technique charts to be effective. First, the radiographic equipment for which the charts are developed must be calibrated.

Calibration ensures that the kVp, milliamperage (mA), and exposure time settings are accurate. Second, all of the film processors must be comparable in their performance for producing the proper radiographic density and contrast. Poor radiographic quality could result from inconsistencies in processing or from the radiographic equipment being out of calibration, rather than the improper selection of exposure factors. A good quality control program on all radiographic equipment will monitor any variability in the equipment's performance.

Practical Tip

Equipment Performance

Radiographic equipment must be operating within normal limits for technique charts to be effective.

Accurate measurement of part thickness is a critical condition for the effective use of technique charts. The measured part thickness determines the selected kVp and mAs values for the radiographic examination. If the part is measured inaccurately, incorrect exposure factors may be selected. It is imperative that measurement of part thickness be standardized throughout the radiology department.

Practical Tip

Measurement of Part Thickness

Accurate measurement of part thickness is critical to the effective use of exposure technique charts.

Calipers are devices that measure part thickness and should be easily accessible in every radiographic room (Figure 9-1). In addition, the technique chart should specify the exact location for measuring part thickness. Part measurement may be performed at the location of the CR midpoint or the thickest portion of the area to be radiographed. Errors in part thickness measurement are one of the more common mistakes made when consulting technique charts.

DESIGN CHARACTERISTICS

Technique charts can vary widely in terms of their design, but they share some common characteristics. The primary exposure factors of kVp, mA, and exposure time, and common accessory devices used such as film-screen type and grid ratio are in-

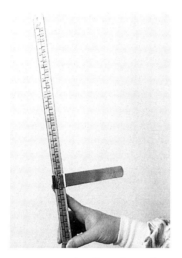

FIGURE 9-1 A caliper is used to measure part thickness. *From Mosby's radiographic instructional series: radiographic imaging, St Louis, 1998, Mosby.*

cluded regardless of the type of technique chart used. The exposure factors that should be standardized in technique charts are listed in Box 9-1.

Box 9-1 *Contents Standardized in a Technique Chart*

Anatomic part	Grid ratio
Automatic exposure control detector selections, if applicable	Kilovoltage peak
	Milliamperage
Central ray location	Part thickness and measuring point
Exposure time	Position or projection
Film-screen combination	Source-to-image receptor distance
Focal spot size	

Types of Technique Charts

Two primary types of exposure technique charts exist: fixed kVp/variable mAs and variable kVp/fixed mAs. Each type of chart has different characteristics, and both have advantages and disadvantages. Technique charts can be differentiated by

TABLE 9-1   EXPOSURE TECHNIQUE CHART CHARACTERISTICS

Design Type	Part Measurement	Contrast Scale	Radiographic Contrast	Patient Dose	Tube Heat Load
Variable kVp/ fixed mAs	Critical	Shorter	Variable	Higher	Increased
Fixed kVp/ variable mAs	Less critical	Longer	Standardized	Lower	Decreased

comparing them on the need for accurate measurement, contrast scale and its variability, patient dose, and heat load on the x-ray tube (Table 9-1).

VARIABLE kVp/FIXED mAs TECHNIQUE CHART

The **variable kVp/fixed mAs technique chart** is based on the concept that kVp can be increased as the anatomic part size increases. Specifically, the baseline kVp is increased by 2 for every 1-cm increase in part thickness, whereas the mAs is maintained (Table 9-2). The baseline kVp is the original kVp value predetermined for the anatomic area to be radiographed. The baseline kVp is then adjusted for changes in part thickness.

Accurate measurement of part thickness is critical to the effective use of this type of technique chart. Part thickness must be measured accurately to ensure that the 2-kVp adjustment is applied appropriately. The radiographer consults the technique chart and prepares the exposure factors specified for the type of radiographic examination (i.e., mAs, SID, grid use, and type of film-screen combination). The anatomic part is measured accurately and the kVp is adjusted appropriately. For example, a standard exposure technique for a patient's knee measuring 10 cm is 63 kVp at 20 mAs, high-speed film-screen combination, and use of a 12:1 table Bucky grid. A patient with a knee measuring 14 cm would then require a change only in the kVp, from 63 to 71 (2 kVp change for every 1-cm change in part thickness).

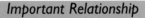
Important Relationship

Variable kVp/Fixed mAs Technique Chart

The variable kVp chart adjusts the kVp for changes in part thickness while maintaining a fixed mAs.

Determining the baseline kilovoltage for each anatomic area has not been standardized. Historically, a variety of methods have been used to determine the baseline kVp value. The goal is to determine a kVp value that will adequately penetrate

TABLE 9-2	VARIABLE KILOVOLTAGE/FIXED mAs TECHNIQUE CHART		

Anatomic part	**Knee**	Film-screen combination	**400 speed**
Projection	**AP**	Table top/Bucky	**Bucky**
Measuring point	**Midpatella**	Grid ratio	**12:1**
Source-to-image receptor distance	**40 inches**	Focal spot size	**Small**

cm	kVp	mAs
10	63	20
11	65	20
12	67	20
13	69	20
14	71	20
15	73	20
16	75	20
17	77	20
18	78	20

the anatomic part when using the 2-kVp adjustment for every 1-cm change in tissue thickness. The baseline kVp value can be determined experimentally with the use of radiographic phantoms.

Developing a variable kVp technique chart that can be used effectively throughout the kilovoltage range has proved problematic. In addition, technologic advances in imaging receptors may challenge the applicability of the variable kVp/fixed mAs type technique chart.

In general, changing the kVp values for changes in part thickness may be ineffective throughout the entire scope of radiographic examinations. A variable kVp/fixed mAs chart may be most effective when small extremities, such as hands, toes, and feet, are being imaged. At this low kVp level, small changes in kVp may be more effective than changing the mAs.

Practical Tip

Applicability of a Variable kVp/Fixed mAs Technique Chart

Variable kVp technique charts may be more effective when small extremities are being imaged.

This type of chart has the advantage of being easy to formulate because exposure changes are easy to make to compensate for different part sizes. However, because kVp is variable, radiographic contrast may vary as well, and these types of charts tend to be less accurate for part size extremes. Adequate penetration of the part is not necessarily assured, and radiographs produced with the use of this type of chart tend to have higher radiographic contrast.

FIXED kVp/VARIABLE mAs TECHNIQUE CHART

The **fixed kVp/variable mAs technique chart** (Table 9-3) uses the concept of selecting an optimal kVp value required for the radiographic examination and adjusting the mAs for changes in part thickness. **Optimal kVp** can be described as the kVp value that is high enough to ensure penetration of the part but not too high to diminish radiographic contrast. For this type of chart, the optimal kVp value for each part is indicated, and mAs is varied as a function of part thickness.

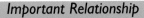

Important Relationship

Fixed kVp/Variable mAs Technique Charts

Fixed kVp/variable mAs technique charts identify optimal kVp values and vary the mAs for changes in part thickness.

TABLE 9-3	**FIXED KILOVOLTAGE/VARIABLE mAs TECHNIQUE CHART**

Anatomic part	**Knee**	Film-screen combination	**400 speed**
Projection	**AP**	Table top/Bucky	**Bucky**
Measuring point	**Midpatella**	Grid ratio	**12:1**
Source-to-image receptor distance	**40 inches**	Focal spot size	**Small**

cm	kVp	mAs
10-13	73	10
14-17	73	20
18-21	73	40

Optimal kVp values required for each anatomic area have not been standardized. Although charts identifying common kVp values for different anatomic areas can be found, experienced radiographers tend to develop their own optimum kVp values. The goal is to determine the kVp that will penetrate the part without compromising radiographic contrast. Specifying the optimal kVp value used in a fixed kVp/variable mAs technique chart encourages all radiographers to adhere to the departmental standards.

Once optimal kVp values are established, fixed kVp/variable mAs technique charts will alter the mAs for the change in thickness of the anatomic part. A general guideline used for mAs changes is for every 4- to 5-cm change in part thickness, the mAs should be adjusted by a factor of 2. Using the previous example for a patient's knee measuring 10 cm and an optimal kVp, the exposure technique would be 73 kVp at 10 mAs, high-speed film-screen in combination with a 12:1 table Bucky grid. A patient with a knee measuring 14 cm would then require a change only in the mAs, from 10 to 20 (a 4-cm increase in part thickness requires a doubling of the mAs).

Accurate measurement of the anatomic part is important but less critical compared with the accuracy needed with variable kVp type charts. An advantage of fixed kVp/variable mAs technique charts is that patient groups can be formed around 4- to 5-cm changes. Patient thickness groups can be created instead of listing thickness changes in increments of 1 cm.

 Practical Tip

Fixed kVp/Variable mAs and Part Measurement

Accuracy of measurement is less critical with fixed kVp/variable mAs technique charts than with variable kVp/fixed mAs technique charts.

The fixed kVp/variable mAs technique chart has the advantages of easier use, more consistency in the production of quality radiographs, greater assurance of adequate penetration of all anatomic parts, standardization of radiographic contrast, and increased accuracy with extreme variances in size of the anatomic part.

Exposure Technique Chart Development

Radiographers can develop effective technique charts that will assist in exposure technique selection. The steps involved in technique chart development are similar regardless of the design of the technique chart. The primary tools needed are radiographic phantoms, calipers for accurate measurement, and a calculator. Once optimal radiographs are produced using these phantoms, exposure techniques can be **extrapolated** (mathematically estimated) for imaging other similar anatomic areas.

A critical component in the technique chart developed is to determine a minimum kVp value that will adequately penetrate the anatomic part to be radiographed. One method available is to use the concept of comparative anatomy. The concept of **comparative anatomy** can assist the radiographer in determining minimum kVp values. This concept states that different parts of the same size can be radiographed using the same exposure factors provided that the minimum kVp value needed to penetrate the part is used in each case. For example, a radiographer knows what exposure factors to use with a particular radiographic unit for a knee that measures 10 cm in the anteroposterior (AP) aspect, but he or she is now confronted with radiographing a shoulder. The radiographer measures the shoulder in the AP aspect and determines that it measures 10 cm. The radiographer does not have a technique for a shoulder for this radiographic unit. The concept of comparative anatomy states that the shoulder in this case can be radiographed successfully using the same technique that the radiographer has for the 10-cm knee as long as the minimum kVp to penetrate the part has been used for the shoulder or knee.

DEVELOPMENT STAGES

The stages for development of exposure technique charts are similar regardless of the type of chart. Patient-equivalent phantoms for sample anatomic areas provide a means for establishing standardized exposure factors. Using the concept of comparative anatomy assists the radiographer in extrapolating exposure techniques for similar anatomic areas. After the initial development of an exposure technique chart, the chart must be tested for accuracy and revised if needed.

The first task is to determine the type of technique chart that will be used in the department. The type of technique chart selected will determine the baseline kVp level. Typically, variable kVp/fixed mAs technique charts use a lower kVp value than fixed (optimal) kVp/variable mAs technique charts.

During initial technique chart development, several phantom radiographs will be produced to demonstrate a range of quality radiographs. All of the radiographs must be reviewed and the radiographs deemed unacceptable according to departmental standards eliminated. The goal is to determine the baseline exposure techniques to be used to produce the quality radiographs.

For variable kVp/fixed mAs technique charts, the remaining acceptable images should provide an upper and lower limit of kilovoltages to be used for the anatomic area. Using the extrapolation technique, the kVp values for changes in part thickness by 1 cm must be determined.

For fixed kVp/variable mAs technique charts, the acceptable radiograph using the highest kVp value should be selected. This radiograph will represent the optimal kVp used for the anatomic area. Using the extrapolation technique, the mAs values for changes in part thicknesses of 4 to 5 cm must be determined. Box 9-2 provides an example.

BOX 9-2 *How to Develop a Fixed kVp/Variable mAs Exposure Technique Chart*

Step 1 Pelvis phantom is positioned on the radiographic table for an anteroposterior (AP) projection of the right hip. The central ray (CR) is at the midpoint of the hip, the source-to-image receptor distance (SID) is 40 inches, and collimation is to film size. The part was measured (26 cm) at the CR entrance point. Select initial exposure technique factors based on departmental standards.

Step 2 Using the kVp/mAs 15% rule, the following five radiographs are produced:

    1. 51 kVp at 200 mAs
    2. 60 kVp at 100 mAs
    3. 70 kVp at 50 mAs
    4. 81 kVp at 25 mAs
    5. 93 kVp at 12.5 mAs

Step 3 Radiographs 1 and 5 are deemed unacceptable.

Step 4 Radiograph 3 is selected as optimum based on departmental standards.

Step 5 The following technique chart is developed by extrapolating the exposure techniques (variable mAs) for changes in part thickness.

Anatomic part	**Hip**	Film-screen combination	**400 speed**
Projection	**AP**	Table top/Bucky	**Bucky**
Measuring point	**CR entrance**	Grid ratio	**12:1**
SID	**40 inches**	Focal spot size	**Small**

cm	kVp	mAs
16-19	70	12.5
20-23	70	25
24-27	70	50
28-31	70	100
32-35	70	200

Box 9-3 lists the development stages for an exposure technique chart.

After the initial development of an exposure technique chart, it must be tested and revised. Poor radiographic quality may result when the exposure technique chart is not used properly. Radiographers need to problem solve through the numerous exposure variables that could have contributed to a poor-quality radiograph before making the assumption the chart is ineffective.

A commitment by management and staff to use exposure technique charts is critical to the consistent production of quality radiographs. Well-developed technique charts are of little use if radiographers choose not to consult them.

> **Box 9-3** *How to Develop an Exposure Technique Chart*
>
> 1. Select a kVp value appropriate to the anatomic area to be radiographed. Determine the mAs value that will produce the desired radiographic density.
> 2. Using a patient-equivalent phantom, produce several radiographs, varying the kVp and mAs values. Use the general rules for exposure technique adjustment (i.e., the 15% rule). Radiographic densities should be similar.
> 3. Evaluate the quality of the radiographs, and eliminate those deemed unacceptable.
> 4. Of the remaining acceptable radiographs, select those having the kVp value appropriate for the type of technique chart desired.
> 5. Extrapolate the exposure techniques (variable kVp or variable mAs) for changes in part thickness.
> 6. Use the concept of comparative anatomy to develop technique charts for similar anatomic areas.
> 7. Test the technique chart for accuracy, and revise if needed.

Review Questions

1. What is defined as *preestablished guidelines used to select standardized exposure factors*?
   A. Comparative anatomy
   B. Extrapolation technique
   C. Exposure technique chart
   D. Automatic exposure control

2. _____ is the primary patient factor that determines the selection of exposure factors.
   A. Age
   B. Part measurement
   C. Physical condition
   D. Weight

3. A primary goal of exposure technique charts is to
   A. extend the life of the x-ray tube.
   B. improve the radiographer's accuracy.
   C. consistently produce quality images.
   D. increase the patient work flow.

4. Which of the following is an important condition required for technique charts to be effective?
   A. Equipment must be calibrated to perform properly.
   B. One technique chart should be used for all radiographic units.
   C. All technologists should use the same mA station.
   D. The chart should not be revised once it has been used.

5. Which of the following factors would *not* be standardized on technique charts?
   A. Milliamperage
   B. Grid ratio
   C. SID
   D. Patient age

6. What type of exposure technique system uses a fixed mAs regardless of part thickness?
  A. Fixed kVp
  B. Variable kVp
  C. Manual
  D. AEC

7. Of the following, which is most important when using a technique chart?
  A. One radiographer revises the chart.
  B. A high mA value is set.
  C. The part is measured accurately.
  D. Patient history is included.

8. What is an advantage of the fixed kVp technique chart?
  A. It produces higher-contrast images.
  B. It reduces patient exposure.
  C. kVp changes are easy to make.
  D. Smaller technique changes are possible.

9. What is a disadvantage of the variable kVp technique chart?
  A. It produces lower-contrast images.
  B. It is difficult to construct.
  C. It may not be effective with small extremities.
  D. It increases heat load on the x-ray tube.

10. In creating either type of exposure technique chart, what is most important?
  A. Achieving adequate penetration of the anatomic part
  B. Selecting the same milliamperage value
  C. Not requiring radiographers to consult them
  D. Producing images with similar radiographic contrast

CHAPTER 10

Automatic Exposure Control

PURPOSE

AEC SYSTEMS
Photomultiplier Tube Systems
Ionization Chamber Systems

LIMITATIONS OF AEC SYSTEMS
Interchangeability of Film-Screen Systems
Minimum Response Time
Lack of Calibration

TECHNICAL CONSIDERATIONS WITH AEC
Centering of the Part
Detector Selection
kVp and mA Selections
Density Selections
Collimation
Backup Time
The Patient
Bucky Selection
mAs Readout

ANATOMIC PROGRAMMING

FILM CRITIQUE

REVIEW QUESTIONS

1 Define all of the key terms in this chapter.

2 State all of the important relationships in this chapter.

3 State the purpose of automatic exposure control (AEC).

4 Describe how photomultiplier tubes and ionization chambers are used are used in AEC systems.

5 Explain each of the limitations of AEC systems.

6 Explain each of the technical considerations to be taken with AEC systems.

7 State what is meant by *anatomic programming* or *anatomically programmed radiography (APR)*.

automatic exposure control (AEC)
detectors
photomultiplier (PM) tube
ionization/ion chamber

minimum response time
backup time
anatomic programming/anatomically
    programmed radiography (APR)

Automatic exposure control (AEC) is one method for setting exposure factors to ensure that a quality radiographic image is produced. When setting a manual (not automatic) technique, the radiographer selects the kilovoltage peak (kVp), milliamperage (mA), and exposure time based on many factors, including source-to-image receptor distance (SID), the thickness and tissue type of the part, the pathology, and the image receptor. A technique chart helps standardize manual techniques. If the radiographer accurately assesses all variables involved in producing the radiograph and the technique chart is accurate, the resulting image should be of optimal quality. However, if the radiographer does not account for (perhaps forgetting to check the SID) or misjudges (maybe not realizing that the patient has a pleural effusion), the resulting image will be suboptimal.

AEC systems are designed to produce radiographs with optimal density by controlling the amount of radiation exposure reaching the film. When used correctly, AEC should produce consistently optimal density radiographs because, based on sensitometry, a specific amount of radiation to the film produces a specific density. If the x-ray exposure is terminated when the exposure corresponding to optimal density is reached, the resultant radiograph should demonstrate optimal density (Figure 10-1).

Important Relationship

X-Ray Exposure and Density

The amount of density on a film depends on the amount of radiation exposure reaching the film. The greater the exposure to the film, the greater the resulting density.

AEC systems must measure the radiation exposure reaching the image receptor; once a preset amount (that which corresponds to optimal density) is reached, the systems shut off the x-ray timer, thereby terminating the radiation. Such a system makes it easier to produce consistent levels of radiographic density. AEC systems have limitations, however. The radiographer must be aware of several technical considerations to use AEC systems successfully. Another type of system, anatomic programming, sometimes is present on the same radiographic units as AEC systems and can assist in the setting of proper exposure factors.

Purpose

AEC systems also are called *automatic exposure devices (AEDs)*, and sometimes they are erroneously referred to as *phototiming*. **Automatic exposure control (AEC)** is a

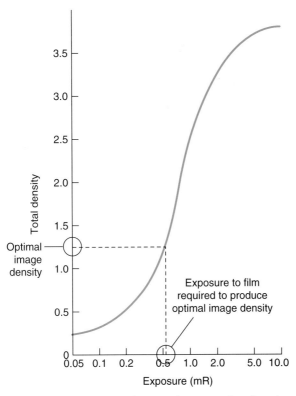

FIGURE 10-1 Sensitometric curve demonstrating the relationship between x-ray exposure at the film level and the resulting radiographic density. A specific amount of x-ray exposure must reach the film to produce optimal image density.

system used to consistently control radiographic density by terminating the length of exposure based on the amount of radiation reaching the image receptor. There are many thousands of possible combinations of kVp, mA, SID, exposure time, film-screen system speeds, and grid ratios. When combined with patients of various sizes and with various pathologic conditions, the selection of proper exposure factors becomes a difficult task. Technique charts make setting technical factors much more manageable, but there are always patient factors that require the radiographer's assessment and judgment. When using AEC systems, the radiographer must still use individual discretion to select an appropriate kVp, mA, film-screen system, and grid. However, the AEC device will determine the exposure time (and therefore total exposure) that is used. AEC is not a panacea, but it can make obtaining optimal radiographic densities significantly less difficult.

Principle of AEC Operation

Once a predetermined amount of radiation is transmitted through a patient, the x-ray exposure is terminated. This determines the exposure time and therefore the resulting density.

AEC Systems

All AEC devices work by the same principle of operation: radiation is transmitted through the patient and converted into an electrical signal, terminating the radiographic exposure. This occurs when a predetermined amount of radiation has been detected, as indicated by the amount of electrical signal that has been produced. The difference in AEC systems lies in the type of device that is used to convert radiation into electricity. Two types of AEC systems have been used: those that use photomultiplier tubes and those that use ionization chambers. Photomultiplier tube systems generally represent the first generation of AEC systems used in radiography, and it is from this type of system that the term *phototiming* has evolved. The term *phototiming* specifically refers to the use of an AEC device that uses photomultiplier tubes, even though these systems are not common today. Therefore the use of the term *phototiming* is usually in error. The more common type of AEC system in use today uses ionization chambers. Regardless of the specific type of AEC system used, almost all systems use a set of three radiation-measuring detectors, arranged in some specific manner (Figure 10-2). The radiographer selects the configuration of these devices, determining which one(s) of the three will actually measure radiation exposure reaching the image receptor. These devices are variously referred to as *sensors, chambers, cells, pick-ups,* or *detectors.* These radiation-measuring devices are referred to here for the remainder of the discussion as **detectors.**

Radiation-Measuring Devices

Detectors are the AEC devices that measure the amount of radiation transmitted. The radiographer selects which of the three detectors will be used.

PHOTOMULTIPLIER TUBE SYSTEMS

A **photomultiplier (PM) tube** is an electronic device that converts visible light energy into electrical energy. Photomultiplier tube AEC devices are considered

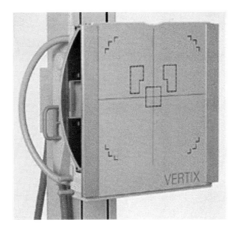

FIGURE 10-2 The size and arrangement of the three AEC detectors are clear on this upright chest stand. *Courtesy Philips Medical Systems.*

exit-type devices because the detectors are positioned behind the cassette (Figure 10-3) so that radiation must exit the cassette before it is measured by the detectors. Light paddles serve as the detectors, and the radiation interacts with the paddles, producing visible light. This light is transmitted to remote PM tubes that then convert this light into electricity. The timer is tripped and the radiographic exposure is terminated when a sufficiently large charge has been received. This electrical charge is in proportion to the radiation to which the light paddles have been exposed. PM tube systems have largely been replaced with ionization chamber systems.

IONIZATION CHAMBER SYSTEMS

An **ionization chamber,** or **ion chamber,** is a hollow cell that contains air and is connected to the timer circuit via an electrical wire. Ionization chamber AEC devices are considered entrance-type devices because the detectors are positioned in front of the cassette (Figure 10-4) so that radiation interacts with the detectors just before interacting with the cassette. When the ionization chamber is exposed to radiation from a radiographic exposure, the air inside the chamber becomes ionized, creating an electrical charge. This charge travels along the wire to the timer circuit. The timer is tripped and the radiographic exposure is terminated when a sufficiently large charge has been received. This electrical charge is in proportion to the radiation to which the ionization chamber has been exposed. Compared with PM tubes, ion chambers are less sophisticated and less accurate, but they are less prone to failure. Most of today's AEC systems use ionization chambers.

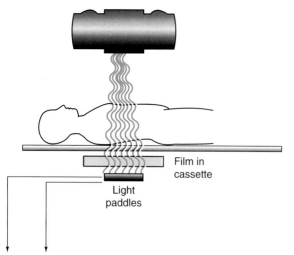

Light paddles, together with photomultiplier tubes, measure radiation exposure after passing through the cassette

FIGURE 10-3 The photomultiplier tube AEC system has the light paddles (detectors) located directly below the cassette. This is an exit-type device in that the x-rays must exit the cassette before they are measured by the detectors.

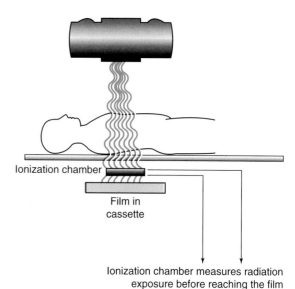

Ionization chamber measures radiation exposure before reaching the film

FIGURE 10-4 The ionization chamber AEC system has the detectors located directly in front of the cassette. This more modern system is termed *entrance-type* in that the x-ray exposure is measured just before entering the cassette.

Important Relationship

Function of the Ionization Chamber

The ionization chamber interacts with transmitted radiation before it reaches the film. Air in the chamber is ionized, and an electric charge that is proportional to the amount of radiation is created.

Limitations of AEC Systems

AEC systems are excellent at producing consistent levels of radiographic density when used properly, but the radiographer should also be aware of some technical limitations of using an AEC system.

INTERCHANGEABILITY OF FILM-SCREEN SYSTEMS

Different film-screen systems cannot be interchanged easily once an AEC device is calibrated to produce specific densities. When a radiographic unit with AEC is first installed, and at intervals thereafter, the AEC device is calibrated. The purpose of calibration is to ensure that consistent and appropriate radiographic densities are produced. When calibration is performed, it is done for a particular film-screen system speed. If the radiographer was to use a different speed of film or screen, the AEC device cannot sense this and instead will produce a density based on the system for which it was calibrated, resulting in a level of density that is either too much or too little. For example, if a 100 speed film-screen system was used with an AEC device instead of the appropriate 400 speed film-screen system, the resulting image will have too little density because the exposure was stopped as preset for the more sensitive 400 speed system. Some radiographic units have AEC devices that can accommodate more than one speed of film-screen system. With these types of units, there is some means of indicating on the control panel which film-screen system will be used for the next exposure.

Practical Tip

Film-Screen Systems and AEC

When an AEC system is used, the radiographer must be certain to use the film-screen system for which the AEC system was calibrated. If more than one film-screen system is used in a department, the radiographer should use the system for which the AEC system was calibrated.

MINIMUM RESPONSE TIME

The term **minimum response time** refers to the shortest exposure time that the system can produce. Minimum response time usually is longer with AEC systems than with other types of radiographic timers. That is, other types of radiographic timers usually are able to produce shorter exposure times than AEC devices. This can be a problem with some segments of the patient population, such as pediatric patients and uncooperative patients. With pediatric patients and others who cannot or will not cooperate with the radiographer by holding still or holding their breath during the exposure as needed, AEC devices may not be the technology of choice.

Practical Tip

Patient Motion and AEC

Because the minimum response time for AEC is longer than that for other types of radiographic timers, the radiographer must decide carefully whether the AEC should be used for particular patients and examinations. If a patient is unable to cooperate in remaining still or holding his or her breath, the use of an AEC device probably is not the best choice. The radiographer should instead set a manual technique rather than use the AEC device to prevent the imaging of patient motion.

LACK OF CALIBRATION

For an AEC device to work properly, the radiographic unit and the AEC device must each be calibrated to accepted standards. Failure to maintain regular calibration of the unit and AEC device will result in radiographs that lack consistent, reproducible, and appropriate density. This ultimately leads to overexposure of the patient and poor efficiency of the imaging department, as well as the possibility of improper interpretation of radiographs.

Practical Tip

Calibration and Unacceptable Radiographs

If radiographs produced in a specific room using an AEC device consistently have too much or too little density, the radiographer should be sure to check the calibration of the AEC system (or have it checked).

Technical Considerations with AEC

In addition to the limitations of AEC devices, radiographers must be aware of some important technical considerations peculiar to AEC systems.

CENTERING OF THE PART

Proper centering of the part being examined is essential when using an AEC system. The area of radiographic interest must be centered properly over the detector(s) that the radiographer has selected. Improper centering of the part over the selected detector(s) produces a radiograph that is either underexposed or overexposed. For example, when an AEC device is used for a lateral lumbar spine image, if the central ray is too far posterior and the center detector is selected (as appropriate), the soft tissue will superimpose the detector rather than the spine. In this case the soft tissue behind the spine will demonstrate optimal density, but the spine itself will be underexposed (Figure 10-5). Inaccurate centering is probably the most common cause of suboptimal density when AEC is used.

DETECTOR SELECTION

Selection of the detector(s) to be used for a particular examination is critical when using an AEC system. The selected detectors actively measure radiation during exposure. It is important to measure radiation that passes through the anatomic area of radiographic interest. The general guideline is to select the detector(s) that will be superimposed by the anatomic structures that are of greatest interest and

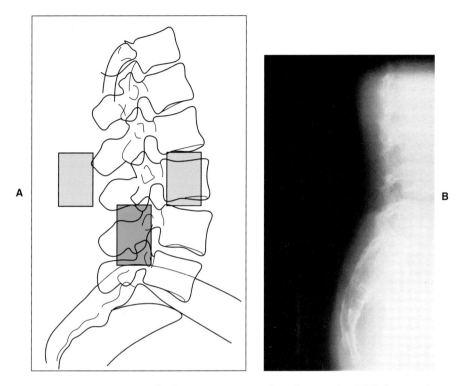

FIGURE 10-5 Centering the key anatomic area directly over the AEC detector is critical in producing optimal density radiographs. Whatever anatomic area is located over the detector will have optimal density. **A,** With the center detector selected, the centering for this lateral lumbar spine is posterior to the lumbar vertebral bodies. The lamina, spinous processes, and soft tissue cover the detector. **B,** The resulting radiograph demonstrates appropriate density just posterior to the vertebral bodies, but the bodies themselves are underexposed. This radiograph is unacceptable because of inaccurate centering.

need to be visualized on the radiograph. Failure to use the proper detectors results in a radiograph that is either underexposed or overexposed. In the case of a posteroanterior (PA) chest radiograph, the area of radiographic interest includes the lungs and heart; therefore one or two outside detectors should be selected to place the detectors directly beneath the critical anatomic part. If the center detector were mistakenly selected, the anatomy superimposing this detector includes the thoracic spine. If the exposure is made, the resultant image will demonstrate optimal density in the spine, with the lungs overexposed (Figure 10-6). In the manual that accompanies the radiographic unit, manufacturers of AEC devices provide recommendations for which detectors to use for specific examinations. Recommendations for detector selection also can be found in many radiographic procedures textbooks.

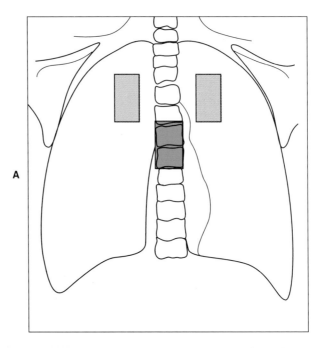

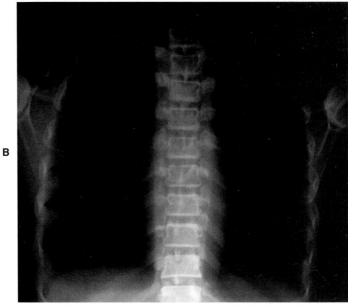

FIGURE 10-6 Selecting the detector(s) to be located directly under the critical anatomic area may make the difference between an optimal and unacceptable image. The posteroanterior (PA) chest should be imaged using both outside detectors to locate them directly under the lung tissue. **A,** This diagram shows that the center detector was inappropriately selected for the PA chest, placing the thoracic spine directly over the detector. **B,** The resulting chest radiograph demonstrates optimal density in the area of the spine, but the lung fields are notably overexposed.

Accurate Part Centering and Detector Selection

Accurate centering and detector selection are critical with AEC systems because the radiograph will demonstrate optimal density of the anatomy located directly over the detector. If the area of radiographic interest is not directly over the selected detector, that area probably will be overexposed or underexposed.

kVp AND mA SELECTIONS

In that AEC controls only the radiographic density and has no effect on radiographic contrast, the kVp for a particular examination should be selected as it would be for that examination regardless of whether an AEC device is used. The radiographer must select the kVp value that provides appropriate scale of contrast and is at least the minimum to penetrate the part. In addition, the higher the kVp value used, the shorter the exposure time needed by the AEC device. Because high kVp radiation is more penetrating (reducing the total amount of x-ray exposure to the patient because more x-ray photons exit the patient) and the detectors are measuring quantity of radiation, the preset amount of radiation exposure is reached sooner with high kVp. Overall, the kVp selected should be high enough to produce the radiographic contrast appropriate to the part being examined while keeping the patient's exposure as low as possible.

AEC, kVp, and Radiographic Contrast

Assuming the radiographer is selecting or using a kVp value above the minimum needed to penetrate the part, adjusting this value will not affect density when using an AEC device. It will affect radiographic contrast, however (Figure 10-7). The radiographer must be sure to set the kVp value as needed to ensure adequate penetration and to produce the appropriate scale of contrast.

When the radiographer uses a control panel that allows the mA and time to be set independently, he or she should select the mA value as it would be for that particular examination regardless of whether an AEC device is used. The mA value selected will have a direct effect on the exposure time needed by the AEC device. Therefore, if the radiographer wants to decrease exposure time for a particular examination, this may be accomplished easily by increasing the mA value. Increasing or decreasing the mA value will not affect the image density but will have a definite impact on the length of the exposure.

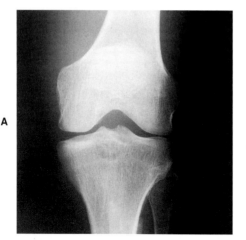 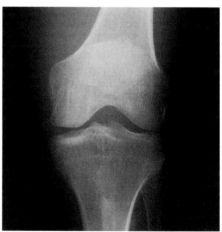

A

B

FIGURE 10-7 Adjustment of kVp with AEC examinations does not affect image density but does affect contrast. Both knees were imaged using the center detector, and all other factors were identical, except for the kVp value. **A,** Imaged at 55 kVp, this knee demonstrates a short scale of contrast. **B,** Imaged at 90 kVp, this image has a much longer scale of contrast, but the density remains essentially the same.

DENSITY SELECTIONS

AEC devices are equipped with density controls that allow the radiographer to fine-tune the radiographic density that will be produced by the unit. These generally are in the form of buttons on the control panel that are numbered −2, −1, +1, and +2. The actual numbers presented on density controls vary, but each of these buttons will change exposure time by some predetermined amount or increment expressed as a percentage. A common increment that is used is 25%, meaning that the predetermined exposure level needed to terminate the timer can be either increased or decreased from normal in one increment (+25% or −25%) or two increments (+50% or −50%). Manufacturers usually provide information for their equipment on how these density controls should be used. Common sense and practical experience should also serve as guidelines for the radiographer.

Practical Tip

AEC and Density Settings

Routinely using plus or minus density settings to produce acceptable radiographs indicates that a problem exists, possibly a problem with the AEC device.

COLLIMATION

Collimation is a factor when using AEC systems because the additional scatter radiation produced by collimation left too open may cause the detector to terminate the exposure prematurely. The detector is unable to distinguish transmitted radiation from scattered radiation and, as always, ends the exposure when a preset amount of exposure has been reached. In that the detector is measuring both types of radiation exiting the patient, the timer is turned off too soon when scatter is excessive, resulting in underexposure of the area of interest. The radiographer should open the collimator to the extent that the part being radiographed will be imaged appropriately, but not so much as to cause the AEC device to stop the exposure before the area being imaged is exposed properly.

BACKUP TIME

Backup time refers to the maximum length of time the x-ray exposure will continue when using an AEC system. The backup time may be set by the radiographer or controlled automatically by the radiographic unit. It may be set as backup exposure time or as backup mAs (the product of mA and exposure time). The role of the backup time is to act as a safety mechanism when an AEC system fails or the equipment is not used properly. In either case, the backup time protects the patient from receiving unnecessary exposure and protects the x-ray tube from reaching or exceeding its heat loading capacity.

Important Relationship

Function of Backup Time

Backup time, the maximum exposure time allowed during an AEC examination, serves as a safety mechanism when the AEC is not used or is not functioning properly.

The backup time might be reached as the result of operator oversight when an AEC examination, such as a chest x-ray study, is done at the upright Bucky and the radiographer has set the control panel for table Bucky. The table detectors will have to wait an enormous time to measure enough radiation to terminate the exposure. In a case such as this, the backup time limits the patient's exposure and keeps the tube from overloading.

When controlled by the radiographer, the backup time should be set high enough to be greater than the exposure needed but low enough to protect the patient from excessive exposure in case of a problem. Setting the backup time at 150% to 200% of the expected exposure time is appropriate. If the backup timer is periodically or routinely being used to terminate the exposure, higher mA values should be used to shorten the exposure time.

Important Relationship

Setting Backup Time

Backup time should be set at 150% to 200% of the expected exposure time. This allows the properly used AEC system to appropriately terminate the exposure but protects the patient and tube from excessive exposure if a problem occurs.

THE PATIENT

Some patients may require greater technical consideration when an AEC device is used for their radiographic procedures. Abdominal examinations using AEC devices can be compromised if a patient has an excessive amount of bowel gas. If a detector is superimposed by an area of the abdomen with excessive gas, the timer will terminate the exposure prematurely, resulting in an underexposed radiograph. Likewise, destructive pathologic conditions can cause underexposure of the area of radiographic interest. The presence of positive contrast media, an additive pathologic condition, or a prosthetic device superimposing the detector can cause excessive density.

The size, shape, and location of the anatomic area of interest also affects the use of AEC systems. If the area of radiographic interest does not completely cover the detector (e.g., the clavicle), the resulting density may be inappropriate. In addition, if the detector must be very close to the edge of the patient's body (e.g., shoulder or pediatric chest), it is important that the detector be covered completely by the anatomic part of interest. If a portion of the detector is exposed directly by the x-ray beam, the radiation exposure level required to terminate the exposure will be reached almost immediately, resulting in underexposure of the area of interest.

Important Relationship

The Patient and AEC

When an AEC device is used, if the anatomic area directly over the detector does not represent the anatomic area of radiographic interest, inappropriate density may result. This can happen when the anatomic area over the detector contains a foreign object, a pocket of air, or contrast media or if the anatomic area does not cover the detector completely.

The radiographer must consider these circumstances individually and determine how best to image the patient. Using the density control buttons may work in some cases, whereas in others it may be necessary to recenter the patient. Sometimes, the best solution is to set a manual technique using a technique chart. An AEC device is not a replacement for a knowledgeable radiographer using critical thinking skills.

Bucky Selection

Many radiographic units use AEC devices in both the table Bucky and an upright Bucky. If more than one Bucky per radiographic unit uses AEC, the radiographer must be certain to select the correct Bucky before making an exposure. Failure to do so will result in the patient and film being exposed to excessive radiation. The backup time will be reached and the exposure terminated. This will require that a repeat radiographic study be done, thereby again increasing the patient's dose.

A similar problem can occur when not using a Bucky, such as with cross table, tabletop, or stretcher/wheelchair studies. If the AEC system is activated with these types of examinations, an unusually long exposure will result because the detectors are not being exposed to radiation. As mentioned already, the backup time will probably be reached and the patient's dose excessive. Some radiographic units are designed so that an exposure will not occur if the AEC device has been selected and there is no cassette sensed in the Bucky.

 Practical Tip

AEC and Non-Bucky Studies

The radiographer should be certain to deactivate the AEC system and use a manual technique when doing any radiographic study where the film is located outside of the Bucky.

mAs Readout

When a radiographic study is performed using an AEC device, the total amount of radiation (mAs) required to produce the appropriate density is determined by the system. Many radiographic units include a mAs readout display, where the actual amount of mAs used for that image is displayed immediately after the exposure, sometimes for only a few seconds. It is critical that, when available, the radiographer take note of this information. Knowledge of the mAs readout provides a number of advantages. It allows the radiographer to become more familiar with manual technical factors. If the image is suboptimal, knowing the mAs readout provides a basis from which the radiographer can make exposure adjustments by switching to manual technique. There may be studies with different positions where AEC and manual technique are combined because of difficulty with accurate centering. Knowing the mAs readout for the anteroposterior (AP) lumbar spine gives the radiographer an option to switch to manual technique for the obliques, making technique adjustments based on factual mAs information.

Practical Tip

AEC and mAs Readout

If the radiographic unit has a mAs readout display, the radiographer should be sure to notice what it reads after the exposure is made. This information can be invaluable.

Anatomic Programming

Anatomic programming, or **anatomically programmed radiography (APR),** refers to a radiographic system whereby the radiographer selects a particular button on the control panel that represents an anatomic area and a preprogrammed set of exposure factors is displayed and selected for use. These controls appear differently on different units (Figure 10-8), but all operate on the same principle. APR is controlled by an integrated circuit or computer chip that has been programmed with exposure factors for different projections and positions of different anatomic parts. Once an anatomic part and projection or position has been selected, the radiographer can adjust the exposure factors that are displayed.

APR and AEC are not related in their functions, other than as systems for making exposures. However, these two different systems are commonly combined on radiographic units because of their similar dependence on integrated computer cir-

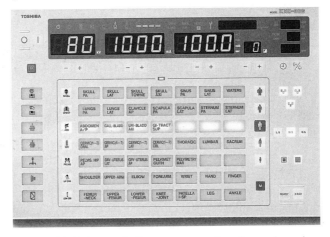

FIGURE 10-8 Anatomically programmed radiography selections are seen on this console. The radiographer can choose from posteroanterior lungs, lateral skull, knee, and hand, among many. Each selection will display the preprogrammed technical factors that the radiographer can decide to use or adjust. *Courtesy Toshiba America Medical Systems.*

cuitry. APR and AEC often are used in conjunction with one another. A radiographer can use APR to select a projection or position for a specific anatomic part and view the kVp, mA, and exposure time for a manual technique that are displayed. The radiographer can then opt to use AEC to determine the exposure time. With some radiographic units, when APR is used in conjunction with AEC, the APR system not only selects and displays manual exposure factors but also selects and displays the AEC detectors to be used for a specific radiographic examination. As is true with AEC, APR is a system that automates some of the work of radiography. However, the individual judgment and discretion of the radiographer is still required to use the APR system correctly in the production of optimal quality radiographs.

 FILM CRITIQUE

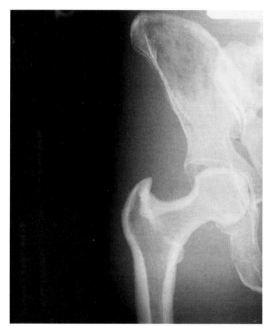

FIGURE 10-9 Image A was produced using 70 kVp, 200 mA, AEC exposure, center detector, 400 speed film-screen combination, and a 40-inch source-to-image receptor distance.

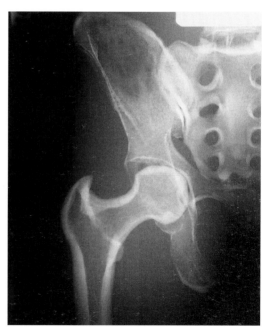

FIGURE 10-10 Image B was produced using 70 kVp, 200 mA, AEC exposure, center detector, 400 speed film-screen combination, and a 40-inch source-to-image receptor distance.

1. Evaluate each radiograph and discuss its quality.

2. For each image, evaluate its exposure variables and discuss their effect on the quality of the image (regardless of whether it is apparent on the radiograph).

3. For each image, identify any adjustments that could be made in the exposure factors to produce an optimal image?

Review Questions

1. The purpose of AEC is to control
   A. kVp.
   B. mA.
   C. density.
   D. contrast.

2. AEC devices work by measuring
   A. radiation leaving the tube.
   B. radiation that is transmitted through the patient.
   C. radiation that is absorbed by the patient.
   D. attenuation of primary radiation by the patient.

3. How many detectors are usually found in an AEC system?
   A. 1
   B. 2
   C. 3
   D. 4

4. Minimum response time refers to
   A. the proper exposure time needed for an optimal exposure when an AEC device is used.
   B. exposure time minus the amount of time the AEC detectors are measuring radiation.
   C. the difference in exposure times between AEC systems and electronic timers.
   D. the shortest exposure time possible when an AEC device is used.

5. Which of the following statements about AEC examinations is true?
   A. Adjusting the mA value affects image density.
   B. Adjusting the kVp value affects image density.
   C. Adjusting the backup time affects image density.
   D. Adjusting the density controls affects image density.

6. Which one of the following statements comparing ionization chamber AEC systems with photomultiplier (PM) tube systems is true?
  A. Ionization chamber systems are accurately called *phototimers*.
  B. Ionization chamber systems measure radiation before it interacts with the cassette.
  C. PM tube systems are more modern.
  D. PM tube systems measure radiation before it interacts with the cassette.

7. The purpose of the backup timer is to
  A. ensure a diagnostic exposure each time AEC is used.
  B. produce consistent levels of density on all radiographs.
  C. determine what exposure time will be used.
  D. limit unnecessary x-ray exposure.

8. What will happen if AEC is activated for a stretcher chest study?
  A. An inappropriately short exposure will occur.
  B. An inappropriately long exposure will occur.
  C. An appropriate exposure will likely occur.
  D. Underexposure of the radiograph will occur.

9. The purpose of anatomic programming is to
  A. present the radiographer with a preselected set of exposure factors.
  B. override AEC when the radiographer has made a mistake in its use.
  C. determine which AEC detectors should be used for a particular examination.
  D. prevent overexposure and underexposure of radiographs, which sometimes happen when AEC is used.

10. Which one statement concerning both AEC and APR is true?
  A. The skilled use of both requires less knowledge of exposure factors on the part of the radiographer.
  B. The use of both requires the radiographer to be less responsible for accurate centering of the anatomic part.
  C. The individual judgment and discretion of the radiographer is still necessary when using these.
  D. The tasks involved with practicing radiography generally are made more difficult with these systems.

CHAPTER 11

Exposure Factor Modification

PEDIATRIC PATIENTS

PROJECTIONS AND POSITIONS

CASTS AND SPLINTS

Casts
Splints

BODY HABITUS

PATHOLOGIC CONDITIONS

SOFT TISSUE TECHNIQUE

CONTRAST MEDIA

GENERATOR TYPE

REVIEW QUESTIONS

OBJECTIVES

1 Define all of the key terms in this chapter.

2 State all of the important relationships in this chapter.

3 Identify exposure factor modification adjustments for the following patients and equipment variables:
   Pediatric patients
   Anatomic parts in casts and splints
   Contrast media procedures
   Types of x-ray generators
   Soft tissue

4 Describe the relationship between exposure factor selection and anatomic part thickness.

5 Describe how pathologic conditions affect attenuation of the primary x-ray beam.

KEY TERMS

body habitus
contrast medium (media)
positive contrast media

negative contrast media
voltage ripple

Appropriate exposure factor selection is critical to the production of an optimal quality radiograph. The responsibility of creating a quality radiograph lies solely with the radiographer. Thus the radiographer must be able to recognize a multitude of patient and equipment variables, have a thorough understanding of how these variables affect the resulting radiograph, and make adjustments to produce a quality image. This chapter addresses exposure factor modification techniques not mentioned in preceding chapters.

Pediatric Patients

Pediatric patients are a technical challenge for radiographers for a number of reasons, including difficulty in properly setting exposure factors. Pediatric patients, because of their smaller size, require lower values of kilovoltage peak (kVp) and mAs (the product of milliamperage and exposure time) compared with adults. The difficult question becomes "How much less?" Children should not be considered just small adults. Improper exposure, whether overexposure or underexposure, appears to be the leading cause of inadequate radiographs in pediatric patients.

Pediatric chest radiography requires the technologist to choose fast exposure times to stop diaphragm motion in patients who cannot or will not voluntarily suspend their breathing. This fast exposure time eliminates the possibility of using automatic exposure control (AEC) systems for pediatric chest radiography.

 Practical Tip

Pediatric Chest Exposure Time

An exposure time of 0.0083 s (1/120 s) should be used to minimize the appearance of motion on the radiograph.

Table 11-1 displays the minimum kVp values necessary to penetrate the pediatric chest.

TABLE 11-1	MINIMUM kVp VALUES THAT ARE REQUIRED TO PENETRATE THE CHEST IN CHILDREN
Chronological Maturity	**Minimum kVp to Penetrate the Part**
Premature	50
Infant	55
Child	60

Skull radiograph exposure factors used for adults can be used for pediatric patients 6 years of age and older because the bone density of these children has developed to that of an adult. However, exposure factors must be changed for patients younger than 6 years of age. It is recommended that the radiographer decrease the kVp value by at least 15% to compensate for this lack of bone density.

Practical Tip

Pediatric Skull Radiography

The radiographer should decrease the kVp value by 15% from an adult technique for skull radiography when performed on pediatric patients younger than 6 years old.

For all other examinations and anatomic parts of pediatric patients, general rules can be used for determining the proper exposure settings. Recommendations for pediatric techniques as derived from technique charts that have been established for adults are presented in Table 11-2.

Projections and Positions

Different radiographic projections and patient positions of the same anatomic part often require modification of exposure factors. For example, an oblique position of the lumbar spine requires more exposure than an anteroposterior (AP) projection because of an increase in the amount of tissue that the primary beam must pass

TABLE 11-2   ADAPTING EXPOSURE FACTORS FOR CHILDREN BASED ON EXPOSURE FACTORS FOR ADULTS, EXCLUDING CHEST AND SKULL EXAMINATIONS

Age (in years)	Exposure Factor Adaptation
Fixed kVp/Variable mAs Techniques	
0-5	25% of mAs indicated for adults
6-12	50% of mAs indicated for adults
Variable kVp/Fixed mAs Techniques	
0-1	30% of mAs indicated for adults
2-5	60% of mAs indicated for adults
6-9	70% of mAs indicated for adults
10-12	90% of mAs indicate for adults

through (Figure 11-1). However, an oblique position of the ankle and an AP projection of the ankle can be exposed with the same technique because of the similarity in the amount of tissue thickness (Figure 11-2). It should be noted that part thickness measurements are made through the path of the central ray.

A lateral position of the wrist requires more exposure than an AP projection of the same part because of the increase in amount of tissue the primary beam must

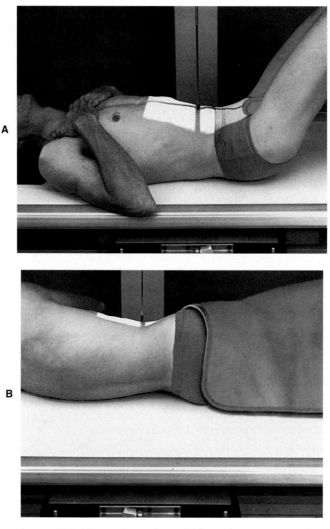

FIGURE 11-1 Comparison of part thickness between anteroposterior **(A)** and oblique lumbar spine positions **(B).** *From Ballinger P:* Merrill's atlas of radiographic positions and radiologic procedures, *ed 9, St Louis, 1999, Mosby.*

pass through (Figure 11-3). However, a lateral position of the humerus and an AP projection of the humerus could be radiographed successfully with the same technique because the amount of tissue is virtually the same (Figure 11-4).

General guidelines can be followed to change exposure factors based on variations in radiographic projection or patient position. For both oblique and lateral patient positions, exposure factors should be changed based on only the increased amount of tissue as compared with the AP projection.

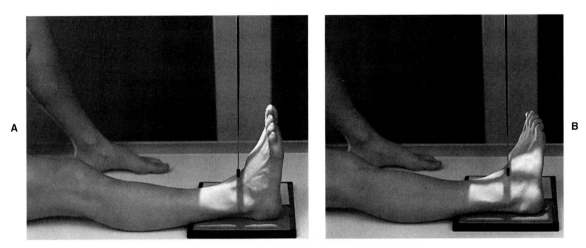

FIGURE 11-2 Comparison of part thickness between anteroposterior **(A)** and oblique **(B)** ankle positions. *From Ballinger P:* Merrill's atlas of radiographic positions and radiologic procedures, *ed 9, St Louis, 1999, Mosby.*

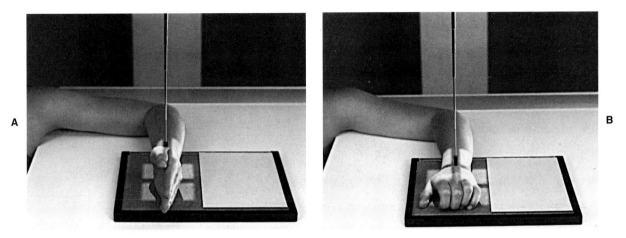

FIGURE 11-3 Comparison of part thickness between **(A)** lateral and **(B)** AP wrist positions. *From Ballinger P:* Merrill's atlas of radiographic positions and radiologic procedures, *ed 9, St Louis, 1999, Mosby.*

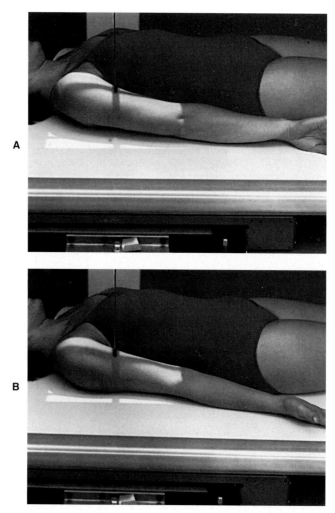

FIGURE 11-4 Comparison of part thickness between lateral **(A)** and anteroposterior **(B)** humerus positions. *From Ballinger P:* Merrill's atlas of radiographic positions and radiologic procedures, *ed 9, St Louis, 1999, Mosby.*

 Practical Tip

Exposure Modification for Changes in Patient Position from AP to Lateral/Oblique Positions

The radiographer should increase the kVp value by 15% (2 × mAs) for each additional centimeter of tissue caused by moving the patient from an AP position to a lateral or oblique position. This increase in kVp will maintain density for the oblique and lateral radiographs.

There is an exception to this rule pertaining to the lateral projection of the lumbar spine. This part of the body is very thick and requires an increase in exposure compared with other examinations.

Practical Tip

Exposure Modification for Lateral Lumbar Spine Radiographs

Part thickness should not be measured through the central ray. The radiographer should measure the AP projection just below the tip of the sternum and the lateral projection at the level of L2. As previously discussed, the kVp value should be increased by 15% (2 × mAs) for each additional centimeter of tissue caused by moving the patient from an AP position to a lateral position.

Casts and Splints

Casts and splints can be produced with materials that attenuate x-rays differently. Selecting appropriate exposure factors can be challenging because of the wide variation of materials used for these devices. The radiographer should pay close attention to both the type of material and how the cast or splint is used.

CASTS

Casts can be produced with either fiberglass or plaster. Fiberglass generally requires no change in exposure factors from the values used for the same anatomic part without a cast.

Practical Tip

Exposure Factor Selection for Fiberglass Casting Materials

Fiberglass casts require no change in exposure factors from the usual technique for that body part.

Plaster, however, presents a problem in terms of exposure factors. It is readily agreed that plaster casts require an increase in exposure factors compared with that needed to radiograph the same part without a cast. However, the method and amount of increase in exposure has not been standardized.

One method of approaching the exposure factor conversion is to consider whether the cast is still wet from application or whether it is dry. This approach states that an increase of 2 times the exposure is needed for a dry plaster cast and an increase of 3 times the exposure is needed for wet plaster casts. However, Gratale, Turner, and Burns suggest that determining exposure factors for a casted limb on the basis of whether the cast is wet is dry is not relevant. Instead, they demonstrate that it is more important to consider the thickness of the cast.[1] Thus exposure factor adjustments made for cast materials may be made based on the part thickness using a technique chart. For example, if an AP ankle measured through the central ray is 8 inches without the cast and 12 inches with the cast, the radiographer simply increases the mAs to that of an ankle measuring 12 inches to obtain an acceptable radiograph.

Practical Tip

Exposure Factor Selection for Plaster Casting Materials

Plaster casts require at least 2 times the mAs (or an increased kVp value by 15%) from the usual technique, but they may require more based on the thickness of the casting material.

SPLINTS

Splints present less of a problem in determining appropriate exposure factors than casts. Inflatable (air) and fiberglass splints do not require any increase in exposure. Wood, aluminum, and solid plastic splints may require that exposure factors be increased, but only if they are in the path of the primary beam. For example, if two pieces of wood are bound to the sides of a lower leg, no increase in exposure is necessary for an AP projection because the splint is not in the path of the primary beam and does not interfere with the radiographic image. Using the same example, however, if a lateral projection is produced, the splint is in the path of the primary beam and interferes with the radiographic imaging of the part. This necessitates an increase of 50% in mAs to produce a properly exposed radiograph.

Practical Tip

Exposure Factor Selection for Splints

If an aluminum, wood, or solid plastic splint is located in the path of the primary beam, mAs must be increased by 50% to produce a quality radiograph.

[1]Gratale P, Turner GW, Burns CB: Using the same exposure factors for wet and dry casts, *Radiol Tech* 57(4):325-329, 1986.

Body Habitus

Body habitus refers to the general form or build of the body, including size. It is important for the radiographer to consider body habitus when establishing techniques. There are four types of body habitus: sthenic, hyposthenic, hypersthenic, and asthenic (Figure 11-5).

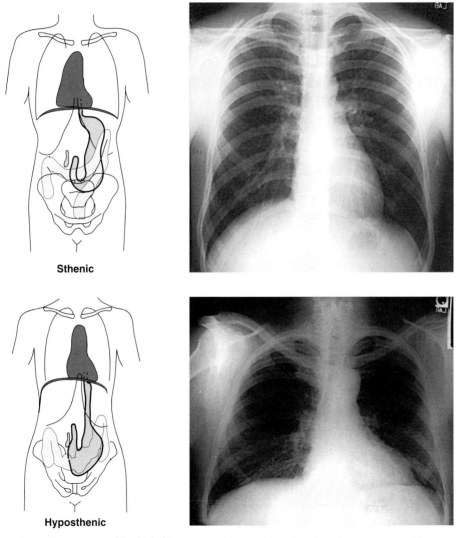

Sthenic

Hyposthenic

FIGURE 11-5 Four types of body habitus. *From Ballinger P:* Merrill's atlas of radiographic positions and radiologic procedures, *ed 9, St Louis, 1999, Mosby.* *Continued*

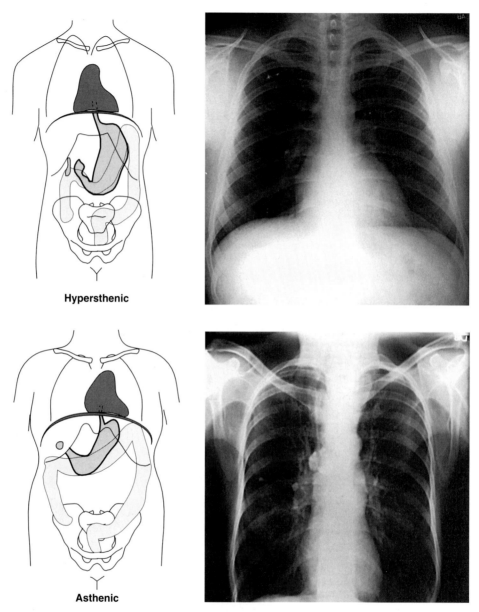

Hypersthenic

Asthenic

FIGURE 11-5, cont'd Four types of body habitus. *From Ballinger P:* Merrill's atlas of radiographic positions and radiologic procedures, *ed 9, St Louis, 1999, Mosby.*

The sthenic body habitus accounts for approximately 50% of the adult population and is commonly called a *normal* or *average* build. Hyposthenic accounts for approximately 35% of adults and refers to a similar type of body habitus as sthenic, but with a tendency toward a more slender and taller build. Together, the sthenic and hyposthenic types of body habitus could, in terms of establishing radiographic techniques, be classified as normal or average of the adult population. This is also convenient because, together, these two types of body habitus account for approximately 85% of adults.

The two remaining types of body habitus are more extreme in terms of size and general occurrence in the adult population. The hypersthenic body habitus, a large, stocky build, accounts for only approximately 5% of adults. These individuals will have thicker part sizes compared with sthenic or hyposthenic individuals, so exposure factors for their radiographic examinations will be higher. *Asthenic* refers to a very slender body habitus and accounts for only 10% of adults. Exposure factors for asthenic individuals will be at the low end of technique charts because their respective part sizes will be thinner than those of sthenic and hyposthenic individuals.

Pathologic Conditions

Technique charts are established without consideration of pathologic conditions. The radiographer must use individual discretion and judgment when preparing to radiograph patients with known or suspected pathologic conditions.

Pathologic conditions that can alter the attenuation of the part being examined are divided into two categories. As described in Chapter 4, additive diseases are diseases or conditions that increase the attenuation of the part, making the part more difficult to penetrate. Destructive diseases are those diseases or conditions that decrease the attenuation of the part, making the part less difficult to penetrate. Table 11-3 presents a list of additive and destructive diseases. Generally speaking, it is necessary to increase kVp when radiographing parts that have been affected by additive diseases and to decrease kVp when radiographing parts that are affected by destructive diseases.

However, it is not necessary to compensate for all additive and destructive diseases. It is often desirable to image diseases with exposure factors that would otherwise normally be used for a specific anatomic part so that the effect of that disease on that part can be visualized clearly. For example, Figure 11-6 demonstrates the first toe radiographed in the AP position. The first metatarsophalangeal joint is affected by osteomyelitis, a destructive disease. It has been radiographed with exposure factors that normally would be used for a toe, without regard for the possible presence of an additive or destructive disease or condition. The normal anatomy of the toe is well visualized, as is the diseased portion.

A similar situation exists with the chest radiograph in Figure 11-7. This patient clearly has pneumonia. The chest was radiographed with exposure factors that normally would be used, without regard for possibility of pneumonia, an additive disease. The radiograph clearly shows properly exposed normal lung tissue, and yet it demonstrates the pneumonia in an excellent manner. Again, it is not always necessary or desirable to compensate exposure factors for additive or destructive diseases before the initial radiograph.

TABLE 11-3   SOME COMMON ADDITIVE AND DESTRUCTIVE DISEASES AND CONDITIONS BY ANATOMIC AREA

Additive Conditions	Destructive Conditions
Abdomen	
Aortic aneurysm	Bowel obstruction
Ascites	Free air
Cirrhosis	
Hypertrophy of some organs (e.g., splenomegaly)	
Chest	
Atelectasis	Emphysema
Congestive heart failure	Pneumothorax
Malignancy	
Pleural effusion	
Pneumonia	
Skeleton	
Hydrocephalus	Gout
Metastases (osteoblastic)	Metastases (osteolytic)
Osteochondroma (exostoses)	Multiple myeloma
Paget's disease	Paget's disease
Osteoporosis	
Nonspecific Sites	
Abscess	Atrophy
Edema	Emaciation
Sclerosis	Malnutrition

In Figure 11-8 an adult chest x-ray is presented. It has been exposed without compensating for pathologic conditions. Free air under the right hemidiaphragm can be seen clearly. This may be clinically significant. An upright abdomen radiograph of the same patient demonstrates the free air in a similar manner. However, the abdomen film should be exposed with about 15% less kVp than normally used for an upright abdomen film because the exposure factors that normally would be used for an upright abdomen would produce a density too dark to easily see the free air.

When it is necessary or desirable to compensate for additive or destructive diseases or conditions, it is best to make changes in kVp only. Changing kVp is funda-

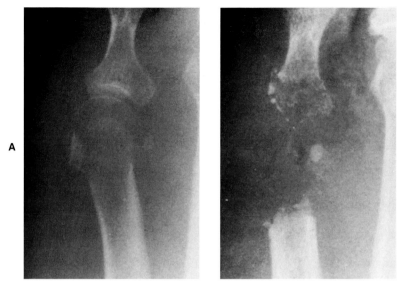

FIGURE 11-6 Radiograph of the first metatarsophalangeal joint demonstrating osteomyelitis. **A,** Soft tissue swelling and periarticular demineralization. **B,** Several weeks later, severe bony destruction. *From Eisenberg R, Dennis C:* Comprehensive radiographic pathology, *ed 2, St Louis, 1995, Mosby.*

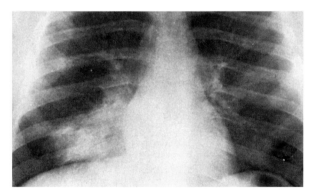

FIGURE 11-7 Radiograph of the chest of a pediatric patient demonstrating pneumonia. *From Eisenberg R, Dennis C:* Comprehensive radiographic pathology, *ed 2, St Louis, 1995, Mosby.*

mentally correct because kVp affects the penetrating ability of the primary beam, and it is the penetrability of the anatomic part that is affected by these particular kinds of diseases or conditions. It is not possible to state an exact amount or percentage of kVp that should be changed because the state or severity of the disease or condition will be different with each patient. However, a minimum change of 15%

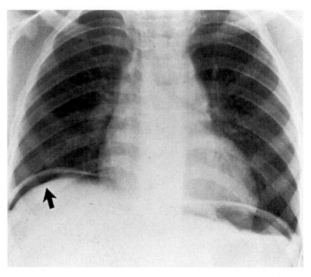

FIGURE 11-8 Radiograph of an adult chest demonstrating free air in the right hemidiaphragm. *From Eisenberg R, Dennis C: Comprehensive radiographic pathology, ed 2, St Louis, 1995, Mosby.*

in kVp is recommended. Disease conditions require changes in exposure factors based on the type and degree of the disease state.

 Practical Tip

Changing kVp to Compensate for Pathologic Conditions

The radiographer should adjust kVp by at least 15% when compensating for pathologic conditions.

Soft Tissue Technique

Objects such as small pieces of wood, glass, or swallowed bones are difficult to visualize radiographically using the normal exposure factors for a particular body part. Several situations in which a soft tissue technique may be needed are visualization of the larynx in a young child with the croup, possible foreign body obstruction in the throat, and foreign body location of the extremities (Figure 11-9). Exposure factors must be altered to demonstrate these soft tissues. In other words, contrast must be increased and overall density must be decreased. To accomplish this, the radiographer decreases kVp. Remember, as kVp is decreased, contrast increases and density decreases if there is no adjustment in mAs.

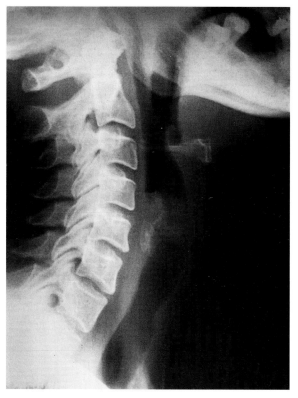

FIGURE 11-9 Lateral soft tissue neck radiograph. *From Ballinger P: Merrill's atlas of radiographic positions and radiologic procedures, ed 9, St Louis, 1999, Mosby.*

 Practical Tip

Changing Exposure Factors to Visualize Soft Tissue

The radiographer should decrease kVp by 15% from the usual technique of the same body part when a soft tissue examination is warranted.

Contrast Media

A **contrast medium** (plural is **media**) is an agent that is introduced into the body to change the attenuation characteristics of a specific anatomic part. Contrast media are categorized as being either positive media or negative media. **Positive contrast media** increase the attenuation characteristics of the part being examined. Barium sulfate and iodine-containing (iodinated) solutions are positive contrast media (Figure 11-10). **Negative contrast media** decrease the attenuation characteristics of the part being examined, such as air and carbon dioxide. Even though negative contrast media decrease the attenuation characteristics of the part being examined, its use does not require a change in exposure factors. Negative contrast media can be used in conjunction with positive contrast media. For example, double-contrast upper gastrointestinal radiography is performed with barium sulfate and pills that dissolve quickly in the stomach to produce carbon dioxide gas (Figure 11-11).

It is readily agreed that contrast media studies require an increase in exposure factors compared with radiographing the same part without contrast media. High kVp (90 and above) is recommended for barium sulfate studies and medium kVp (70 to 80) for procedures requiring iodinated solutions.

Practical Tip

Selection of Exposure Factors for Use with Contrast Media

The radiographer should select a high kVp (90 and above) for barium sulfate studies and a medium kVp (70 to 80) for procedures requiring iodinated solutions.

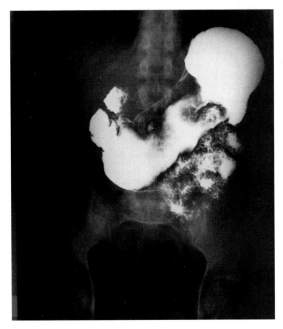

FIGURE 11-10 Radiograph of the abdomen containing positive contrast media.

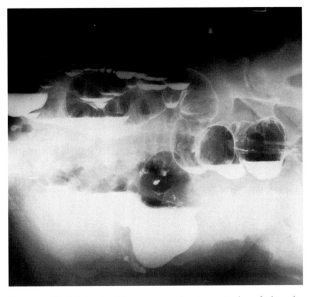

FIGURE 11-11 A double-contrast barium study of the abdomen containing negative contrast media.

Generator Type

The type of x-ray generator that is used with a particular radiographic unit determines, in part, the intensity of the primary beam produced by that unit. Three basic types of x-ray generators are available: single phase, three phase (capable of producing either 6 or 12 pulses per cycle), and high frequency. Each produces a different voltage waveform (Figure 11-12). These waveforms are a reflection of the consistency of the voltage supplied to the x-ray tube during a x-ray exposure. The term **voltage ripple** is used to describe voltage waveforms in terms of the differences in peak voltage. From Figure 11-12 it can be can be seen that for single-phase generation, voltage varies from the peak to a value of 0. Voltage ripple for single-phase generators is said to be 100% because there is total variation in the voltage waveform, from peak voltage to 0 voltage. For three-phase generators, voltage ripple is 13% for 6-pulse, and 4% for 12-pulse. High-frequency generators produce a voltage ripple less than 1%. Voltage input into the x-ray tube is most consistent for high-frequency generators. This information is summarized in Table 11-4.

Generator output must be considered when selecting exposure factors. Some sources present general guidelines concerning changing mAs values to compensate for differences in x-ray generators. Changing mAs will produce the same density on both radiographs but will cause a change in contrast. For example, if a three-phase 12-pulse unit produces a satisfactory radiograph using 80 kVp, 50 mAs, a radiograph with the same density and contrast can be produced on a single-phase unit using 90 kVp, 50 mAs. Density and contrast are maintained because the effective kVp of the single-phase unit is lower than that of the three-phase unit.

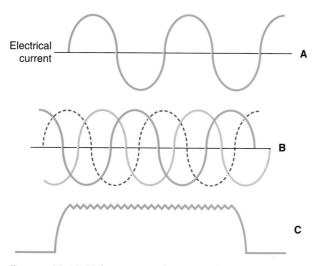

FIGURE 11-12 Voltage wave forms produced by various x-ray generators. **A,** Single phase. **B,** Three phase. **C,** High frequency.

Table 11-4	**Voltage Ripple Occurring from X-Ray Generators**

Type of Generator	Voltage Ripple
Single phase	100%
Three phase, 6 pulse	13%
Three phase, 12 pulse	4%
High frequency	<1%

Ignoring kilovoltage when compensating for generator type will change the scale of contrast because kilovoltage is a controlling factor of radiographic contrast. This became more apparently clear with the advent of high-frequency generators.

Practical Tip

Compensating Exposure Factors for Changing Generator Type

To maintain radiographic density and contrast, the radiographer must decrease the kVp value by 15% for three-phase generators and high-frequency generators compared with single-phase generators.

Separate recommendations for three-phase generators and high-frequency generators are not warranted because the voltage ripple factors are very similar.

Review Questions

1. In determining whether exposure factors should be changed when changing radiographic projections or patient positions, what must be considered?
   A. The presence of either an additive or a destructive disease or condition and the degree to which the attenuating ability of the tissue is changed because of it
   B. The body habitus of the individual patient and whether the patient can achieve the particular position necessary to produce the needed projection or position
   C. Whether the beam must pass through more tissue, less tissue, or the same amount as the previous projection or position
   D. The order in which each radiographic projection or patient position should be produced to avoid excessive changing of exposure factors

2. Which type of splint may require an increase in exposure factors to compensate for the attenuation of the beam by the splint
   A. Air
   B. Aluminum
   C. Inflatable
   D. Fiberglass

3. Positive contrast media
   A. coat the anatomic part they are applied to, requiring an increase in exposure factors.
   B. increase the attenuation characteristics of the parts they are used to examine.
   C. sometimes require an increase in exposure factors and sometimes require a decrease.
   D. are not used by themselves but instead are used in conjunction with negative contrast media.

4. It is most correct to change _____ based on the type of x-ray generator being used.
   A. mA
   B. exposure time
   C. kVp
   D. film-screen system

5. On which two types of body habitus should technique charts be established because they represent about 85% of adults in the population?
   A. Asthenic and hypersthenic
   B. Hyposthenic and hypersthenic
   C. Sthenic and asthenic
   D. Sthenic and hyposthenic

6. If it is determined that a patient has a pathologic disease or condition that can significantly alter the attenuation of the tissues that are affected, the _____ should be changed to compensate for this disease or condition.
   A. mA
   B. exposure time
   C. kVp
   D. film-screen system

7. A patient has possibly swallowed a small chicken bone. The physician requests a lateral view of the cervical spine. How would you change exposure factors to best visualize the soft tissues of the neck?
   A. Increase mAs 2 times.
   B. Decrease mAs 2 times.
   C. Increase kVp by 15%.
   D. Decrease kVp by 15%.

CHAPTER 12

Computed Radiography

DIGITAL FLUOROSCOPY

LIMITATIONS OF CONVENTIONAL RADIOGRAPHY

COMPUTED VERSUS CONVENTIONAL RADIOGRAPHY

Similarities
Differences

COMPUTED RADIOGRAPHY IMAGE CHARACTERISTICS

COMPUTED RADIOGRAPHY IMAGING PROCESS

Image Acquisition
Image Processing
Image Display

DIGITAL IMAGE QUALITY

Resolution
Density
Contrast
Noise

DIRECT RADIOGRAPHY

DIGITAL COMMUNICATION NETWORKS

REVIEW QUESTIONS

OBJECTIVES

1 Define all of the key terms in this chapter.

2 State all of the important relationships in this chapter.

3 Recognize modalities that currently use digital imaging.

4 List the additional equipment needed for digital fluoroscopy.

5 State the limitations of conventional radiography.

6 Compare and contrast conventional and computed radiography techniques.

7 Explain the three-step imaging process in computed radiography.

8 Discuss the primary factors controlling image quality in computed radiography.

KEY TERMS

digital imaging
imaging plate (IP)
postprocessing image enhancement
matrix
pixel

voxel
histogram
algorithms
window level
window width

Advancements in computer technology since the 1970s have made digital imaging a reality in diagnostic radiography. Although the terminology has not yet been standardized, **digital imaging** is defined as an image constructed from numerical data. Different processes are available to obtain digital images. Digital fluoroscopy and computed radiography are both currently used methods that are discussed in this chapter.

Digital imaging is not new to the radiation sciences. Since the introduction of computed tomography (CT) in the 1970s, digital imaging has become standard in several modalities, such as magnetic resonance imaging (MRI), nuclear medicine, and sonography. Each of these modalities has specialized equipment to create images that can be displayed, manipulated, and stored as digital or numerical data.

Digital Fluoroscopy

Digital fluoroscopy has been easily introduced into the radiology department because it can readily be adapted to the image-intensification systems currently used. The fluoroscopic image is obtained in a manner similar to that of conventional fluoroscopy. The exit radiation is absorbed by the input phosphor, converted to electrons, sent to the output phosphor, released as visible light, and then converted to a an electronic video signal for transmission to the television monitor.

In digital fluoroscopy (Figure 12-1), an analog-to-digital converter (ADC) is used to convert the analog (continuous) video signal to digital (numeric) data. The image

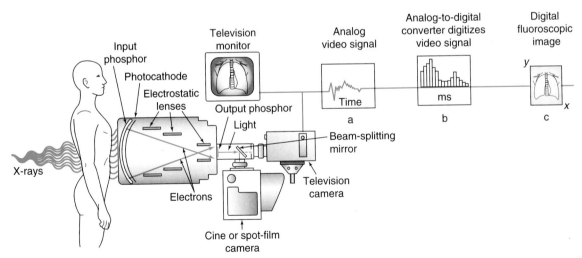

Figure 12-1 Analog and digital signals in fluoroscopy. The video signal from the television camera is analog, where the voltage signal varies continuously. This analog signal is sampled (*a*), producing a stepped representation of the analog video signal (*b*). The numerical values of each step are stored (*c*), producing a matrix of digital image data. The binary representation of each pixel value in the matrix is stored and can be manipulated by a computer. The value of each pixel can be mapped to a brightness level for viewing on a CRT or to an optical density for hard copy on film. *Courtesy Eastman Kodak Company.*

is then viewed on a high-resolution video monitor. It is the conversion of the video signal to digital data that creates the opportunity for manipulation of the image in a variety of ways. Discussion about the composition and manipulation of digital images is further explored in the subsequent sections on computed radiography.

Limitations of Conventional Radiography

The conventional film-screen system poses limitations that can be overcome in computed radiography. The radiographic image created following a divergent x-ray beam's (area x-ray beam) attenuation results in the superimposition of anatomic structures. Obtaining multiple projections of an anatomic area will still result in overlying structures that obscure visualization of the area of interest.

Conventional radiography limits the visibility of a wide range of structures within the same anatomic part. An example is the difficulty of visualizing both soft tissue and bony structures within the same image. When an image is taken in the thorax region, the technique must be selected depending on whether the area of interest is the lung fields or the ribs. In addition, the differentiation of soft tissue structures is limited because the attenuation characteristics among the soft tissues are so similar that the range of visible densities (shades of gray) provides poor visualization.

A primary limiting factor of conventional radiography is that once the radiograph has been processed, the image is permanent and further adjustments cannot be made. If the image is too dark or too light, it must be repeated, causing increased patient exposure.

The information contained on the radiograph also is limited to the range of densities recorded on the film that represent the absorption characteristics of the anatomic area. The radiograph does not provide any quantitative information about the attenuation characteristics of the anatomic tissues.

Last, processing time, storage, and archival of radiographs have created undesirable delays and costs. The amount of time it takes to process the film before viewing the radiograph can delay the progress of an examination or the diagnosis. In addition, the cost of storing radiographs and then retrieving them when needed for comparison has become unmanageable.

Although there are different methods of producing digital images, computed radiography has become a commonly used method. Computed radiography has overcome many of the limitations of conventional radiography. Radiographic images can be obtained, processed, stored, and retrieved in a more timely manner. The computed image has the ability to record a wider range of tissues with one exposure, provide quantitative data on the attenuation characteristics of the tissues, and visualize anatomic structures without the overlying structures.

Computed versus Conventional Radiography

Although the computed image can overcome many of the limitations of conventional radiography, they share several similarities.

SIMILARITIES

The type of computed radiography that is becoming more prevalent in radiology departments uses the same x-ray tube and generator system for exposing the patient to an area x-ray beam. The radiographer continues to select the required exposure factors of milliamperage (mA), exposure time, and kilovoltage peak (kVp). In addition, accurate positioning of the patient for a variety of projections remains a critical part of the imaging process. The imaging receptor, which is similar to a cassette, can be transported easily to distant areas such as the operating room or the patient's bedside. Although the image receptor is different, a latent image will be produced and later processed to form a manifest image.

DIFFERENCES

The differences of computed radiography are key to its overcoming the limitations of conventional radiography.

The imaging receptor is similar to a cassette with an intensifying screen but without radiographic film. This system is sometimes called a *filmless cassette*. In place of the film or screen is an **imaging plate (IP)** that is made of a photostimulable phosphor material that absorbs the photon intensities exiting the patient.

The latent image is formed within this photostimulable phosphor, and the energy is released by a scanning laser beam and then digitized and sent to a computer for processing (Figure 12-2). The photostimulable phosphor is capable of a much wider exposure latitude than conventional radiography. This wide-exposure latitude provides better visualization of soft tissue and bony structures and allows for the adjust-

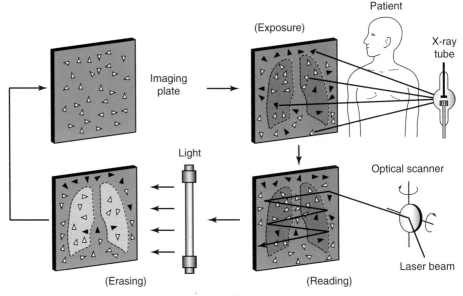

FIGURE 12-2 Principles involved in image recording, reading, and erasing. *Courtesy Fuji Medical Systems.*

ment of either low or high exposure to the imaging plate. The exposed imaging plate is placed in a reader unit or device that will extract the absorbed energy and convert the varying visible light into digital data.

Once the image is converted into digital (numerical) data, the computer can perform **postprocessing image enhancement.** This process allows the manipulation of the image in a variety of ways, such as subtraction, contrast, and edge enhancement.

Computed Radiography Image Characteristics

Unlike a conventional radiograph that is made up of minute strands of black metallic silver, a digital image is displayed as a combination of rows and columns, called a **matrix.** The smallest component of the matrix is the **pixel** (picture element). Each pixel corresponds to a specific region on the imaging plate and represents the x-ray intensity at that location. A numeric value representing a shade of gray is stored for each pixel. This shade of gray is viewed as brightness on a cathode-ray-tube (CRT) or video monitor. "The brightness in each pixel is represented by a long list of digital numbers; each number represents the intensity of a pixel, and the number's location in the list represents the pixel's location in the image."[1] The location of the pixel within the image matrix corresponds to an area within the patient or volume of tissue called **voxel** (Figure 12-3).

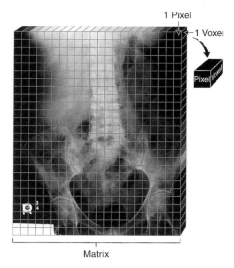

FIGURE 12-3 The location of the pixel within the image matrix corresponds to an area within the patient or volume of tissue, called *voxel.*

[1]Kuni C: *Introduction to computers & digital processing in medical imaging,* Chicago, 1988, Year-Book Medical Publishers.

In computed radiography the size of the matrix needed to produce images of acceptable quality is 1024 × 1024, whereas a matrix size of 2048 × 2048 is preferred. A matrix size of 1024 × 1024 has 1,048,576 individual pixels, whereas a matrix size of 2048 × 2048 has 4,194,304 pixels. Image quality is improved with a larger matrix size having a greater number of pixels (Figure 12-4).

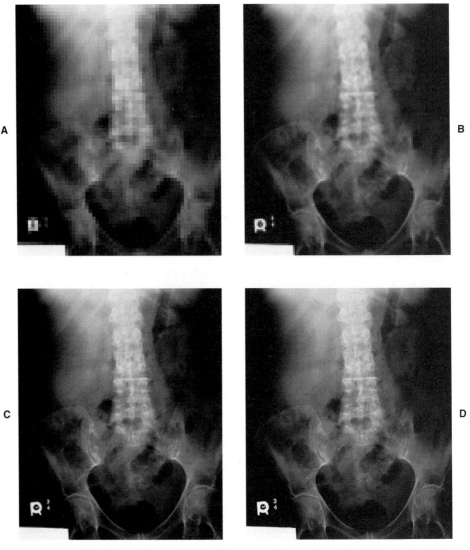

FIGURE 12-4 The larger the matrix size the greater the number of individual pixels. Increasing the number of pixels will improve the quality of the image. **A,** Matrix size is 64 × 64. **B,** Matrix size is 215 × 215. **C,** Matrix size is 1024 × 1024. **D,** Matrix size is 2048 × 2048.

Important Relationship

Matrix Size and Image Quality

Increasing the matrix size increases the number of pixels, thereby increasing the quality of the image. Decreasing the matrix size decreases the number of pixels, thereby decreasing the quality of the image.

Computed Radiography Imaging Process

Three primary stages are involved in computed radiography: image acquisition, image processing, and image display.

IMAGE ACQUISITION

The radiation exiting the patient interacts with the imaging plate, where the photon intensities are absorbed by the photostimulable phosphor. The phosphor consists of barium fluorohalide crystals coated with europium. Although some of the absorbed energy is released as visible light (luminescence), as in conventional radiography, a sufficient amount of energy is stored in the phosphor to produce a latent image. The latent image is formed within the crystals of the photostimulable phosphor following the transfer of energy by a photoelectric effect.

Although the imaging plate can store the absorbed energy for several hours, it is important for the latent image to be processed in a timely manner; otherwise, the stored energy will fade along with the latent image.

The exposed imaging plate is placed in a reader unit that converts the analog image into a digital image for computer processing (Figure 12-5). Once in the reader unit, the imaging plate is scanned with a helium-neon laser beam to release the stored energy as visible light (Figure 12-6). A photomultiplier tube (PMT) collects, amplifies, and converts the light to an electrical signal proportional to the range of energies stored in the imaging plate. The varying electrical signals are sent to the ADC for conversion into digital data. The digitized x-ray intensities or pixels are patterned in the computer to form the image matrix. The image matrix is a digital composite of the varying x-ray intensities exiting the patient (Figure 12-7). Each pixel has a brightness level representing the attenuation characteristic of the volume of tissue imaged.

Before the imaging plate is stored for later use, the plate is scanned with an intense light to release any residual energy that could affect future exposures. Photostimulable phosphors can be reused and are estimated to have a life of 10,000 readings before they need to be replaced.

IMAGE PROCESSING

During image processing, the digital data are evaluated and manipulated before being displayed. The digital data are used to construct a **histogram,** or graphic display,

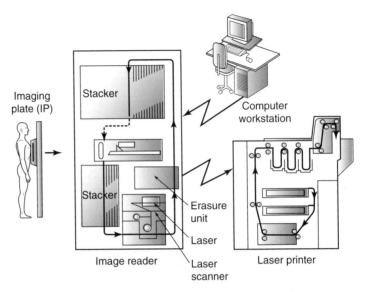

FIGURE 12-5 The exposed imaging plate is place in a reader unit to release the stored image, convert the analog image to a digital image, and send the data to a computer monitor and or a laser printer for a hard copy. The reader unit also erases the exposed imaging plate in preparation for the next exposure. *Courtesy Fuji Medical Systems.*

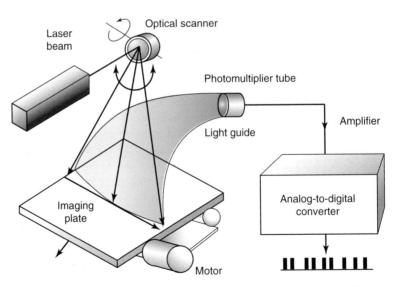

FIGURE 12-6 A neon-helium laser beam scans the exposed imaging plate to release the stored energy as visible light. The photomultiplier tube collects, amplifies, and converts the light to an electrical signal. The analog-to-digital converter converts the analog data to digital data. *Courtesy Fuji Medical Systems.*

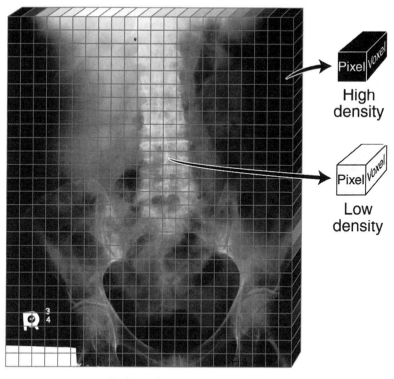

FIGURE 12-7 Each pixel represents a volume of tissue imaged.

of the distribution of pixel values (Figure 12-8). Each image has its own histogram, and it is evaluated to determine the adequacy of the imaging plate exposure to x-rays. If the histogram suggests a low or high exposure, the PMT will adjust the electrical signal accordingly to compensate for the error.

Manufacturers of computed radiography systems have different methods of indicating the x-ray exposure. Each type of system specifies the expected range of x–ray exposure sufficient to produce a quality image. A number is placed on the processed image to indicate the level of x-ray exposure received to the imaging plate. It is important for the radiographer to consider the indicated value because exposure errors will affect the quality of the digital image. If the value indicates a low x-ray exposure to the imaging plate, the PMT increases the electrical signal to adjust for the error. If the value indicates a high x-ray exposure, the PMT suppresses the electrical signal to adjust for the error. Although computed radiography offers the advantage of correcting for exposure errors, image quality can be sacrificed. X-ray exposure errors greater or lesser than 50% will produce poorer-quality images.

Processing **algorithms,** or mathematical formulas, are used to formulate image construction for the specific type of examination performed, such as chest, extremity, spine, or abdomen. The radiographer must indicate the correct radiographic

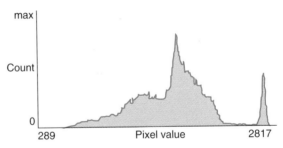

FIGURE 12-8 Histogram showing the number of each of the pixel values in an image. The pixel values (grays) are represented by the horizontal axis; the total number of each pixel value is reflected on the vertical axis. *From Cesar LJ: Computed radiography: its impact on radiographers, J ASRT 68(3), 1997.*

procedure so that the appropriate algorithm will be performed. If the incorrect processing algorithm is selected, the resulting image will not be constructed properly.

IMAGE DISPLAY

Once the image has been processed in a digital format, it can be displayed on a CRT, printed on film, sent to a distant location, or stored on a magnetic or optical disk.

CRT or Video Monitor

When the computed image is displayed on a CRT (soft-copy viewing), it can be manipulated in a variety of ways. The following are four common postprocessing techniques:

1. *Subtraction* (Figure 12-9) is a technique that can remove superimposed structures so the anatomic area of interest is more visible. Because the image is in a digital format, the computer can subtract selected brightness values that will create an image without superimposing structures.

2. *Contrast enhancement* (Figure 12-10) is a postprocessing technique that alters the pixel values to display different brightness levels.

3. *Edge enhancement* (Figure 12-11) is a postprocessing technique that improves the visibility of small, high-contrast structures.

4. *Black/white reversal* (Figure 12-12) is a postprocessing technique that reverses the gray scale from the original radiograph.

One of the factors that has limited the rapid introduction of computed radiography into radiology departments has been the display of images on a CRT. Standard

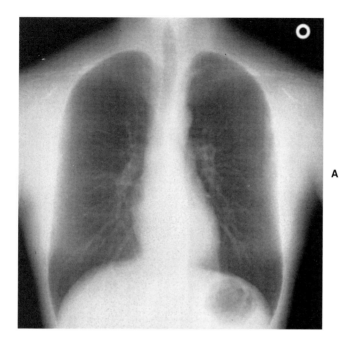

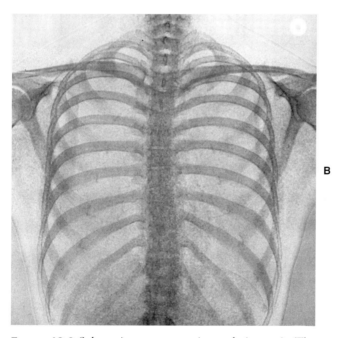

FIGURE 12-9 Subtraction postprocessing techniques. **A,** The skeletal areas are removed. **B,** The lungs and soft tissue are removed.

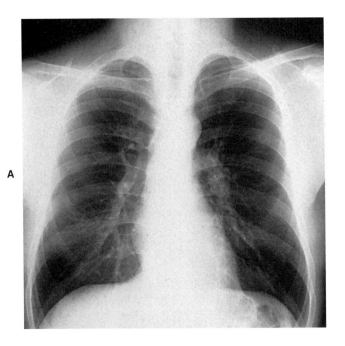

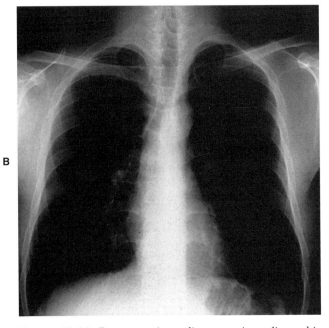

FIGURE 12-10 Postprocessing adjustment in radiographic contrast. **A,** A longer-scale contrast typical of chest radiography. **B,** Contrast has been adjusted to present a higher scale.

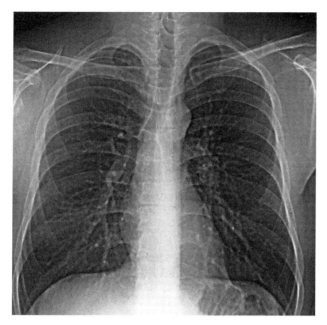

FIGURE 12-11 Radiographic image demonstrates an edge enhancement postprocessing technique.

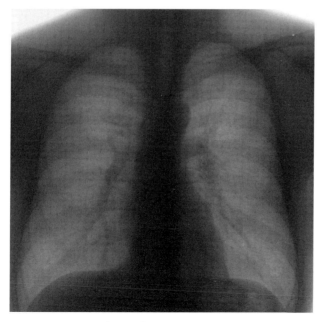

FIGURE 12-12 Radiographic image demonstrates a black/white reversal postprocessing technique.

monitors used in fluoroscopy have a 525-line system. Visualizing a computed image of similar quality to a conventional image requires that the display monitor have high spatial resolution (recorded detail) capabilities. This can be achieved only with monitors that are at least 1000-line systems. The cost associated with installing high-resolution monitors in all locations that would benefit from this technology has been somewhat prohibitive.

Laser Camera Printing

As in conventional radiography, standard hard-copy viewing of images is still common. Computed images can be altered while viewed on a CRT and then printed onto film by a laser camera. Multiple images can be printed on a single sheet, and multiple copies of images postprocessed differently can be printed.

Digital Image Quality

Evaluating the quality of digital images shares many of the same properties as in conventional radiography. Resolution, density, and contrast are all attributes important in the production of quality radiographic images.

RESOLUTION

Spatial resolution and spatial detail are properties of digital imaging comparable to the geometric properties (recorded detail) of conventional radiographic imaging.

Although digital imaging technology has been available since the 1970s, a limiting factor has been its low image resolution. Recent improvements in the imaging plate, reader unit, and display monitors have contributed to the improved resolution of digital images, although computed radiographic images continue to have less resolution than conventional radiography. Transforming data of a continuous form (analog) to a discrete form (digital) results in the loss of some accuracy of information. Conventional radiography has the capability of resolving approximately 6 to 10 Lp/mm (line pairs per millimeter), whereas computed radiography is limited to approximately 2.5 Lp/mm. The resolving capabilities of computed radiography continue to improve.

Resolution also is sacrificed during x-ray absorption by the photostimulable phosphor, laser scanning to extract the absorbed energy, and the ADC.

A major factor in the level of spatial resolution of computed images is the matrix size. As mentioned previously, the greater the number of pixels in a matrix image, the smaller their size. An image made up of a greater number of pixels will provide improved spatial detail.

Pixel Number and Spatial Detail

Increasing the number of pixels in the image matrix increases the spatial detail.

The capabilities of the device used for image viewing also affect the resolution of spatial detail. As discussed, the CRT or video monitor has been a limiting factor in the widespread use of computed radiography. High-resolution monitors of 1000 lines have improved the image display. More recent recommendations are for a CRT monitor to have 2000 lines.

DENSITY

Visualizing anatomic structures within the area of interest on a conventional radiograph requires that the optical density fall within the straight-line region of the sensitometric curve. When optical densities fall outside this region, the density is either too dark or too light, usually resulting in a repeat radiographic study being necessary. Because computed radiography provides wider-exposure latitude, the margin of error for the exposure technique in obtaining densities that will provide sufficient visualization of the anatomic area of interest is greater.

When a sensitometric curve for computed radiography and conventional film are compared, the response of computed images is linear as opposed to the standard S shape (Figure 12-13). This means the imaging plate can respond to exposures that

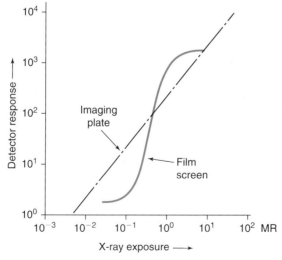

FIGURE 12-13 The imaging plate has wider-exposure latitude compared with conventional film.

vary more greatly than conventional film. In addition, having access to a wider range of densities can improve the visualization of anatomic structures that differ greatly in composition.

The beam that exits the patient contains more than 1000 shades of gray. The visual range of humans is limited to fewer than 32 shades of gray. The processed digital image is only a small sample of the total information contained within the computer.

The **window level** sets the midpoint of the range of densities visible in the image. Changing the window level on the CRT monitor allows the image brightness to be increased or decreased throughout the range of densities (Figure 12-14).

Important Relationship

Window Level and Image Brightness

A direct relationship exists between window level and image brightness on the CRT monitor. Increasing the window level increases the image brightness; decreasing the window level decreases the image brightness.

Adjusting the window level for image brightness on the CRT monitor has the opposite effect on the image density printed for a hard copy. Increasing the window level on the CRT image (increased brightness) decreases the density on the hard-copy film, whereas decreasing the window level on the CRT image (decreased brightness) increases density on the hard copy.

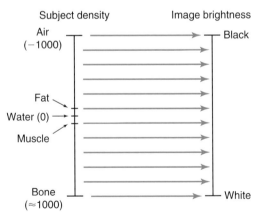

FIGURE 12-14 Changing the window level increases or decreases the image brightness throughout the range of densities recorded in the image. *From Kuni C,* Introduction to computers and digital processing in medical imaging, *Chicago, 1988, Year-Book Medical Publishers.*

CONTRAST

Many of the same principles used to vary contrast in conventional radiography are applicable to computed radiography. Kilovoltage remains the primary exposure factor used to manipulate the radiographic contrast. The kilovoltage should be selected based on the penetration needed, but more important, it should be selected to produce the level of contrast (high or low) needed to best visualize the anatomic area of interest. Because the imaging plates used in computed radiography are more sensitive to scatter radiation, it is recommended to limit the kVp to 80 or less.

Many of the factors used in conventional radiography to control or limit the amount of scatter radiation reaching the film are also used in computed radiography. Grids typically are used with smaller anatomic structures to limit the amount of scatter reaching the imaging plate. In addition, appropriate collimation is used to reduce the amount of scatter interacting with the imaging plate.

Once the computed image is processed, radiographic contrast can be adjusted further to vary visualization of the area of interest. The **window width** is a control that adjusts the radiographic contrast (Figure 12-15). Because the digital image can display densities ranging from -1000 (black) to $+1000$ (white), the display monitor can vary the range or number of densities visible on the image. Adjusting the range of densities visible varies the scale of contrast. When the entire range of densities is displayed (wide window width), the image will have lower contrast, or more shades of gray; when a smaller range of densities is displayed (narrow window width), the image will have higher contrast, or fewer shades of gray (Figure 12-16).

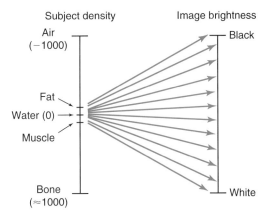

FIGURE 12-15 Changing the window width increases or decreases the range of densities visible. A narrow window width decreases the range of densities and increases contrast. A wider window width increases the range of densities and reduces contrast. *From Kuni C,* Introduction to computers and digital processing in medical imaging, *Chicago, 1988, Year-Book Medical Publishers.*

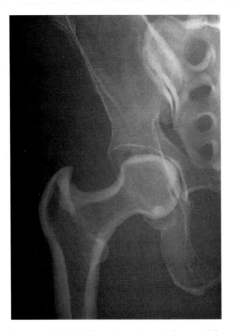 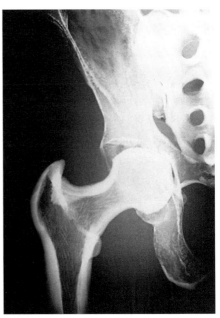

FIGURE 12-16 Changing the window width varies the scale of contrast visible on the computed image.

Important Relationship

Window Width and Radiographic Contrast

A narrow window (decreased) width increases radiographic contrast, whereas a wider window (increased) width decreases radiographic contrast.

This concept is similar to conventional radiography regarding scale of contrast. In conventional radiography, radiographic contrast is inversely related to the range of visible densities. A high-contrast radiograph (few shades of gray) will display a smaller (narrow) range of densities, whereas a lower-contrast radiograph (many shades of gray) will display a greater (wider) range of visible densities.

In computed radiography, an inverse relationship also exists between window width and image contrast.

NOISE

Image noise contributes no useful diagnostic information and serves only to detract from the quality of the image. As in conventional radiography, quantum mottle is the primary source of noise in computed radiography and it is photon dependent.

Quantum mottle is visible as density fluctuations on the image. The fewer photons reaching the imaging plate to form the image, the greater the quantum mottle visible on the digital image.

Important Relationship

Number of Photons and Quantum Mottle

Decreasing the number of photons reaching the imaging plate increases the amount of quantum mottle within the image; increasing the number of photons reaching the imaging plate decreases the amount of quantum mottle within the image.

As mentioned previously, during image acquisition, the PMT can adjust for low or high x-ray exposures. When the x-ray exposure to the imaging plate is too low (decreased number of photons), the density can be corrected but the image shows increased quantum mottle or image noise.

System noise results during the digital imaging process and is not dose dependent. The processes of image acquisition, phosphor conversion fluctuations, laser-beam scanning, and ADC all result in system noise. System noise usually is less of a problem than quantum mottle.

Finally, image noise is more noticeable with the postprocessing techniques of contrast and edge enhancement. All of these sources of image noise contribute no useful information and only degrade the quality of the digital image.

The quality of the computed or digital image depends on many of the same factors as conventional radiography. Density and contrast are affected by the amount of x-ray exposure to the imaging plate, as is the quantum mottle or image noise. In addition to the effect of exposure factors, accurate positioning of the part and proper alignment of the part x-ray beam and imaging plate also affect the quality of the image. The positioning and alignment factors have a greater effect on the quality of the image than in conventional radiography during manual exposure. Similar to using the automatic exposure device (AEC), the resultant image can be affected when the part is not positioned properly or not aligned to the correct photocell. "If the part, beam, and plate are misaligned in such a way that the exposure does not match the algorithm assumptions for that part, the data will not be properly processed to yield an image with expected density and contrast."[2]

Direct Radiography

Further developments in digital imaging will continue as advancements occur in computer technology. One such development is direct radiography. The concept of

[2]Burns C: Using computed digital radiography effectively, *Semin Radiol Tech* 1(1):24-36, 1993.

direct radiography is similar to computed radiography in that specialized detectors receive the exit radiation and the computer generates the initial image. Direct radiography is a system of digital imaging that excludes the ADC step. The system uses specialized equipment to capture the exit x-rays and convert them to electrical signals to create the digital image, thereby eliminating the loss of information during the image acquisition stage.

Currently, the major disadvantage of direct radiography is that the entire radiographic system needs to be replaced. This system is not adaptable to currently used x-ray tubes and generators as is computed radiography. As radiology moves toward complete digital imaging and communication, direct radiography will become more feasible.

Digital Communication Networks

Computed radiography, like CT and MRI, is a method of digital imaging. Digital communication needs in radiology also include the processing and delivery of patient data and subsequent interpretation of radiologic procedures. The ability to integrate both image and written data simultaneously involves a more complex system. Picture archival and communication systems (PACS) is the computer system for digital imaging; radiology information systems (RIS) and hospital information systems (HIS) are the computer systems for written data. The ability to integrate these systems can be accomplished by networks. A network system links all of these computer systems so that images, patient data, and interpretations can be viewed simultaneously by people at different workstations. Network systems are currently being marketed to meet the demands in the radiation sciences. The issues of interoperability and interfacing of these different computer systems is essential for networking systems to function effectively. Communication among these systems is necessary for radiology to realize the full potential of digital communication.

Review Questions

1. What is a limitation of conventional radiography?
   A. Poor resolution
   B. Poor soft tissue differentiation
   C. Increased quantum mottle
   D. Transporting cassettes

2. Computed radiography has the advantage of
   A. less expensive equipment.
   B. improved resolution.
   C. latent image formation.
   D. wide-exposure latitude.

3. What occurs when the exit radiation interacts with a photostimulable imaging plate?
   A. Fluorescence
   B. Energy absorption
   C. Phosphorescence
   D. Photoemission

4. The geometric properties of a computerized image are known as
   A. sharpness.
   B. noise.
   C. mottle.
   D. spatial detail.

5. Image brightness on a CRT is adjusted by
   A. scanning lines.
   B. window level.
   C. window width.
   D. matrix size.

6. Radiographic contrast on a CRT is adjusted by
   A. scanning lines.
   B. window level.
   C. window width.
   D. matrix size.

7. Image noise can be decreased by
   A. decreasing x-ray dose
   B. increasing edge enhancement
   C. increasing x-ray dose
   D. decreasing window level

8. Increasing the window width of a computed image on a CRT will
   A. decrease the brightness.
   B. increase the brightness.
   C. decrease the contrast.
   D. increase the contrast.

9. The smallest component of a matrix image that represents an x-ray intensity is called
   A. pixel.
   B. histogram.
   C. voxel.
   D. brightness.

10. The mathematical formula used to construct a digital image is called a(n)
    A. histogram.
    B. algorithm.
    C. postprocessing enhancement.
    D. matrix.

Summary of Important Relationships

Chapter 1: Radiation and Its Discovery

THE DUAL NATURE OF X-RAY ENERGY

X-rays act both like waves and like particles. (See p. 6.)

WAVELENGTH AND FREQUENCY

Wavelength and frequency are inversely related. If one increases, the other decreases. (See p. 7.)

Chapter 2: The X-Ray Beam

THE FILAMENT

The filament is the source of electrons during x-ray production. (See p. 14.)

FOCUSING THE ELECTRON STREAM

The negatively charged focusing cup condenses the stream of electrons flowing from the cathode and focuses, or directs, it to the anode. (See p. 14.)

THE TARGET

The target is the part of the anode that is struck by the focused stream of electrons coming from the cathode. The target stops the electrons and thus creates the opportunity of the production of x-rays. (See p. 15.)

TUNGSTEN

Because tungsten has a high atomic number (74) and a high melting point (3370° F), it efficiently produces x-rays. (See p. 16.)

DISSIPATING HEAT

As the target rotates and heat within the tube increases, the anode conducts heat to the insulating oil that surrounds the x-ray tube. (See p. 17.)

ROTATING ANODES

Rotating anodes can withstand greater heat loads than stationary anodes because their rotating motion causes a greater physical area, or focal track, to be exposed to electrons. (See p. 18.)

THE PRODUCTION OF X-RAYS

As electrons strike the target, their kinetic energy is transferred to the tungsten atoms in the anode to produce x-rays. (See p. 20.)

INTERACTIONS THAT PRODUCE X-RAY PHOTONS

Bremsstrahlung interactions and characteristic interactions both produce x-ray photons. (See p. 20.)

BREMSSTRAHLUNG INTERACTIONS

Most x-ray interactions in the diagnostic energy range are bremsstrahlung. (See p. 20.)

THERMIONIC EMISSION

When the tungsten filament gains enough heat *(therm)*, the outer-shell electrons *(ions)* of the filament atoms are boiled off, or *emitted*, from the filament. (See p. 24.)

TUBE CURRENT

Electrons flow in only one direction in the x-ray tube—from cathode to anode. This flow of electrons is called the *tube current* and is measured in milliamperes (mA). (See p. 26.)

ENERGY CONVERSION IN THE X-RAY TUBE

As electrons strike the anode target, approximately 99% of their kinetic energy is converted to heat, whereas only approximately 1% is converted to x-rays. (See p. 26.)

KILOVOLTAGE AND THE SPEED OF ELECTRONS

The speed of the electrons traveling from the cathode to the anode increases as the kilovoltage applied across the x-ray tube increases. (See p. 28.)

THE SPEED OF ELECTRONS AND THE QUALITY OF THE X-RAYS

The speed of the electrons in the tube current determines the quality or energy of the x-rays that are produced. The quality or energy of the x-rays that are produced determines the penetrability of the primary beam. (See p. 28.)

kVp AND BEAM PENETRABILITY

As kVp increases, beam penetrability increases; as kVp decreases, beam penetrability decreases. (See p. 28.)

MILLIAMPERAGE, TUBE CURRENT, AND X-RAY QUANTITY

The quantity of electrons in the tube current and quantity of x-rays produced are directly proportional to the milliamperage. (See p. 29.)

EXPOSURE TIME, TUBE CURRENT, AND X-RAY QUANTITY

The quantity of electrons that flows from cathode to anode and the quantity of x-rays produced are directly proportionate to the exposure time. (See p. 30.)

THE QUANTITY OF ELECTRONS, X-RAYS, AND mAs

The quantity of electrons flowing from the cathode to the anode and the quantity of x-rays produced are directly proportionate to mAs. (See p. 30.)

LINE FOCUS PRINCIPLE

The effective focal spot size decreases as the target angle decreases. (See p. 31.)

THE ANODE HEEL EFFECT

X-rays are more intense on the cathode side of the tube. The intensity of the x-rays decreases toward the anode side. (See p. 31.)

LOW-ENERGY PHOTONS, PATIENT DOSE, AND IMAGE FORMATION

Low-energy photons contribute only to patient dose and not to image formation. (See p. 33.)

HEAT UNITS

The number of HUs produced depends on the type of x-ray generator used and the exposure factors selected. (See p. 36.)

Chapter 3: Radiographic Image Formation

DIFFERENTIAL ABSORPTION AND IMAGE FORMATION

A radiographic image is created by passing an x-ray beam through the patient and interacting with an image receptor, such as a film-screen system. The variations in absorption and transmission of the exiting x-ray beam will structurally represent the anatomic area of interest. (See p. 43.)

X-RAY PHOTON ABSORPTION

During attentuation of the x-ray beam, the photoelectric effect is responsible for total absorption of the incoming x-ray photon. (See p. 43.)

X-RAY BEAM SCATTERING

During attenuation of the x-ray beam, the incoming x-ray photon may lose energy and change direction as a result of the Compton effect. (See p. 44.)

IMAGE DENSITIES

The range of image densities are created by the variation in x-ray absorption and transmission as the x-ray beam passes through anatomic tissues. (See p. 46.)

Chapter 4: Radiographic Image Quality

mAs, QUANTITY OF RADIATION, AND RADIOGRAPHIC DENSITY

As the mAs is increased, the quantity of radiation is increased and radiographic density is increased. As the mAs is decreased, the quantity of radiation is decreased and radiographic density is decreased. (See p. 55.)

MILLIAMPERAGE AND EXPOSURE TIME

Milliamperage and exposure time have an inverse relationship when maintaining the same mAs. (See p. 56.)

KILOVOLTAGE AND RADIOGRAPHIC DENSITY

Increasing the kilovoltage peak increases the quantity of radiation reaching the image receptor and therefore increases radiographic density. Decreasing the kilovoltage peak decreases the quantity of radiation reaching the image receptor and therefore decreases radiographic density. (See p. 58.)

SID AND RADIOGRAPHIC DENSITY

As SID increases, radiographic density decreases as a result of the square of the distance. As SID decreases, the radiographic density increases as a result of the square of the distance. (See p. 60.)

SID AND mAs

Increasing the SID requires that mAs be increased to maintain density, and decreasing the SID requires a decrease in mAs to maintain density. (See p. 61.)

GRIDS AND RADIOGRAPHIC DENSITY

Adding, removing, or changing a grid requires an adjustment in mAs to maintain radiographic density. (See p. 62.)

FILM-SCREEN SYSTEM SPEED AND RADIOGRAPHIC DENSITY

The greater the speed of the film-screen system, the greater the amount of density produced on the radiograph; the lower the speed of the film-screen system, the less density produced on the radiograph. (See p. 63.)

FILM-SCREEN SYSTEM SPEED AND mAs

Increasing the film-screen speed requires a decrease to be made to the mAs to maintain density, and decreasing the film-screen speed requires an increase to be made to the mAs to maintain density. (See p. 63.)

PART THICKNESS AND RADIOGRAPHIC DENSITY

A thick anatomic part decreases the radiographic density. A thin anatomic part increases radiographic density. (See p. 64.)

KILOVOLTAGE AND RADIOGRAPHIC CONTRAST

High kilovoltage creates more densities but with fewer differences, resulting in a low-contrast (long-scale) image. Low kilovoltage creates fewer densities but with greater differences, resulting in a high-contrast (short-scale) image. (See p. 70.)

KILOVOLTAGE, SCATTER RADIATION, AND RADIOGRAPHIC CONTRAST

Increasing kilovoltage increases the amount of scatter radiation produced and decreases radiographic contrast. Decreasing the kilovoltage decreases scatter production and reduces the amount of fog, therefore increasing radiographic contrast. (See p. 71.)

SCATTER RADIATION AND RADIOGRAPHIC CONTRAST

Whenever the amount of scatter radiation reaching the image receptor is reduced, the radiographic contrast is increased (higher contrast). (See p. 75.)

FOCAL SPOT SIZE AND RECORDED DETAIL

As focal spot size increases, unsharpness increases and recorded detail decreases; as focal spot size decreases, unsharpness decreases and recorded detail increases. (See p. 79.)

SID, UNSHARPNESS, AND RECORDED DETAIL

Increasing the SID decreases the amount of unsharpness and increases the amount of recorded detail in the image, whereas decreasing the SID increases the amount of unsharpness and decreases the recorded detail. (See p. 81.)

OID, UNSHARPNESS, AND RECORDED DETAIL

Increasing the OID increases the amount of unsharpness and decreases recorded detail, whereas decreasing the amount of OID decreases the amount of unsharpness and increases the recorded detail. (See p. 82.)

INTENSIFYING FILM-SCREEN SPEED, RECORDED DETAIL, AND UNSHARPNESS

Increasing the relative speed of the intensifying film-screen system decreases the recorded detail and increases the amount of unsharpness recorded in the image. Decreasing the relative speed of the intensifying film-screen system increases the recorded detail and decreases the amount of unsharpness recorded in the image. (See p. 85.)

MOTION AND RECORDED DETAIL

Motion of the tube, patient or part, or image receptor greatly decreases recorded detail. (See p. 87.)

OID AND SIZE DISTORTION

As OID increases, size distortion (magnification) increases; as OID decreases, size distortion (magnification) decreases. (See p. 89.)

SID AND SIZE DISTORTION

As SID increases, size distortion (magnification) decreases; as SID decreases, size distortion (magnification) increases. (See p. 90.)

Chapter 5: Scatter Control

COLLIMATION AND PATIENT DOSE

As collimation increases, field size decreases; therefore patient dose also decreases. As collimation decreases, field size increases; therefore patient dose increases. (See p. 103.)

BEAM RESTRICTION, SCATTER CONTROL, AND CONTRAST

Beam restriction reduces the amount of scatter radiation produced, thus increasing radiographic contrast. (See p. 103.)

COLLIMATION AND SCATTER RADIATION

As collimation increases, the field size decreases and the intensity of scatter radiation decreases; as collimation decreases, the field size increases and the intensity of scatter radiation increases. (See p. 104.)

COLLIMATION AND RADIOGRAPHIC CONTRAST

As collimation increases, radiographic contrast increases; as collimation decreases, radiographic contrast decreases. (See p. 104.)

COLLIMATION AND RADIOGRAPHIC DENSITY

As collimation increases, radiographic density decreases; as collimation decreases, radiographic density increases. (See p. 105.)

SCATTER RADIATION AND IMAGE QUALITY

Scatter radiation adds unwanted density to the radiograph and decreases image quality. (See p. 113.)

GRID RATIO AND RADIOGRAPHIC CONTRAST

As grid ratio increases, radiographic contrast increases; as grid ratio decreases, radiographic contrast decreases. (See p. 114.)

FOCUSED VERSUS PARALLEL GRIDS

Focused grids have lead lines that are angled to approximately match the divergence of the primary beam. Thus focused grids allow more transmitted photons to reach the image receptor than parallel grids. (See p. 115.)

GRID FOCAL DISTANCE AND GRID CUTOFF

To eliminate the production of grid cutoff, the radiographer should use an SID within the focal range labeled on the grid. (See p. 117.)

GRID RATIO AND RADIOGRAPHIC DENSITY

As grid ratio increases, radiographic density decreases; as grid ratio decreases, radiographic density increases. (See p. 119.)

GRID RATIO AND PATIENT DOSE

As grid ratio increases, patient dose increases; as grid ratio decreases, patient dose decreases. (See p. 122.)

GRID RATIO AND GRID CUTOFF

As grid ratio increases, the likelihood of grid cutoff increases; as grid ratio decreases, the likelihood of grid cutoff decreases. (See p. 123.)

UPSIDE DOWN FOCUSED GRIDS AND GRID CUTOFF

Placing a focused grid upside down on the image receptor causes a plus density (dark) strip down to appear down the center of the radiograph. (See p. 123.)

LATERAL DECENTERING AND GRID CUTOFF

Angling the x-ray tube across the grid lines or angling the grid itself during exposure produces an overall decrease in density on the radiograph. (See p. 125.)

DISTANCE DECENTERING AND GRID CUTOFF

Using an SID outside of the focal range creates a loss of density at the periphery of the radiograph. (See p. 126.)

Chapter 6: Image Receptors

SENSITIVITY SPECKS AND LATENT IMAGE CENTERS

Sensitivity specks serve as the focal point for development of latent image centers. After exposure, these specks trap the free electrons and then attract and neutralize the positive silver ions. After enough silver is neutralized, the specks become a latent image center and are converted to black metallic silver after processing. (See p. 139.)

SILVER HALIDE AND FILM SENSITIVITY

As the number of silver halide crystals increases, film sensitivity or speed increases; as the size of the silver halide crystals increases, film sensitivity or speed increases. (See p. 141.)

SPECTRAL MATCHING AND DENSITY

To best use a film-screen system, the radiographer must match the color sensitivity of the film with the color emission of the intensifying screen. Failure to do so results in suboptimal density. (See p. 142.)

CROSSOVER AND RECORDED DETAIL

When light from one intensifying screen crosses over the film base and exposes the emulsion on the opposite side, loss of recorded detail occurs. Reducing crossover improves recorded detail. (See p. 144.)

SCREENS, PATIENT EXPOSURE, AND RECORDED DETAIL

Compared with direct-exposure radiography, adding intensifying screens reduces patient exposure but also reduces recorded detail. (See p. 145.)

SCREEN SPEED AND LIGHT EMISSION

The faster an intensifying screen, the more light emitted for the same x-ray exposure. (See p. 148.)

SCREEN SPEED AND PATIENT DOSE

As screen speed increases, radiation dose to the patient decreases; as screen speed decreases, radiation dose to the patient increases. (See p. 148.)

SCREEN SPEED AND DENSITY

As screen speed increases, density increases; as screen speed decreases, density decreases. (See p. 149.)

RARE EARTH PHOSPHORS AND SPEED

Rare earth phosphors are significantly faster than calcium tungstate because of increased absorption and conversion efficiency. (See p. 150.)

PHOSPHOR THICKNESS, CRYSTAL SIZE, AND SCREEN SPEED

As the thickness of the phosphor layer increases, the speed of the intensifying screen increases; as the size of the phosphor crystals increases, the speed of the screen increases. (See p. 151.)

SCREEN SPEED AND RECORDED DETAIL

With any given phosphor type, as screen speed increases, recorded detail decreases, and as screen speed decreases, recorded detail increases. (See p. 153.)

Chapter 7: Radiographic Processing

PRODUCING RADIOGRAPHIC DENSITIES

The developing agents are responsible for reducing the exposed silver halide crystals to metallic silver, visualized as optical densities. Phenidone is responsible for creating the lower densities, and hydroquinone is responsible for creating the higher densities. Their combined effect results in the range of densities visible on the radiograph. (See p. 165.)

CLEARING THE UNEXPOSED CRYSTALS

The fixing agent, ammonium thiosulfate, is responsible for removing the unexposed crystals from the emulsion. (See p. 167.)

ARCHIVAL QUALITY OF RADIOGRAPHS

Maintaining the archival (long-term) quality of radiographs requires that most of the fixing agent be removed (washed) from the film. Staining or fading of the permanent image results when too much thiosulfate remains on the film. (See p. 168.)

ARCHIVAL QUALITY OF RADIOGRAPHS

Permanent radiographs must retain moisture of 10% to 15% to maintain archival quality. Excessive drying can cause the emulsion(s) to crack. (See p. 169.)

REPLENISHMENT AND SOLUTION PERFORMANCE

The replenishment system provides fresh chemistry to the developing and fixing solutions to maintain their chemical activity and volume when depleted during processing. (See p. 173.)

RECIRCULATION AND SOLUTION PERFORMANCE

Recirculation of the developer and fixer solutions is necessary to maintain solution activity and the required agitation. (See p. 178.)

DEVELOPER TEMPERATURE AND RADIOGRAPHIC QUALITY

Variations in developer temperature adversely affect the quality of the radiographic image. Increasing developer temperature increases the density, and decreasing developer temperature decreases the density. Radiographic contrast also may be adversely affected by changes in the developer temperature. (See p. 178.)

MOISTURE AND ARCHIVAL QUALITY

The dryer assembly controls the amount of moisture removal to maintain the archival quality of radiographic film. (See p. 180.)

Chapter 8: Sensitometry

LIGHT TRANSMITTANCE AND OPTICAL DENSITY

As the percentage of light transmitted decreases, the optical density increases; as the percentage of light transmitted increases, the optical density decreases. (See p. 198.)

OPTICAL DENSITY AND LIGHT TRANSMITTANCE

For every 0.3 change in optical density, the percentage of light transmitted has changed by a factor of 2. A 0.3 increase in optical density results from a decrease in the percentage of light transmitted by half, whereas a 0.3 decrease in optical density results from an increase in the percentage of light transmitted by a factor of 2. (See p. 198.)

LOG RELATIVE EXPOSURE

A 0.3 change in log of exposure represents a change in intensity of radiation exposure by a factor of 2. An increase of 0.3 log of exposure results in a doubling of the amount of radiation exposure, whereas a decrease in 0.3 log of exposure results in halving the amount of radiation exposure. (See p. 200.)

FILM SPEED AND OPTICAL DENSITY

For a given exposure, as the speed of a film increases, the optical density produced also increases; as the speed of a film decreases, the optical density decreases. (See p. 202.)

FILM SPEED AND SPEED EXPOSURE POINT

The lower the speed exposure point, the faster the film speed; the higher the speed exposure point, the slower the film speed. (See p. 203.)

SLOPE AND FILM CONTRAST

The steeper the slope of the straight-line region (more vertical), the higher the film contrast; the lesser the slope (less vertical), the lower the film contrast. (See p. 206.)

AVERAGE GRADIENT AND FILM CONTRAST

The greater the average gradient, the higher the film contrast; the lower the average gradient, the lower the film contrast. (See p. 208.)

EXPOSURE LATITUDE AND FILM CONTRAST

Exposure latitude and film contrast have an inverse relationship. High-contrast radiographic film will have narrow latitude, and low-contrast film will have wide latitude. (See p. 209.)

Chapter 9: Exposure Factor Selection

EXPOSURE TECHNIQUE CHARTS AND RADIOGRAPHIC QUALITY

A properly designed and used technique chart standardizes the selection of exposure factors to help the radiographer produce consistent quality radiographs while minimizing patient exposure. (See p. 216.)

VARIABLE kVp/FIXED mAs TECHNIQUE CHART

The variable kVp chart adjusts the kVp for changes in part thickness while maintaining a fixed mAs. (See p. 220.)

FIXED kVp/VARIABLE mAs TECHNIQUE CHARTS

Fixed kVp/variable mAs technique charts identify optimal kVp values and vary the mAs for changes in part thickness. (See p. 222.)

Chapter 10: Automatic Exposure Controls

X-RAY EXPOSURE AND DENSITY

The amount of density on a film depends on the amount of radiation exposure reaching the film. The greater the exposure to the film, the greater the resulting density. (See p. 230.)

PRINCIPLE OF AEC OPERATION

Once a predetermined amount of radiation is transmitted through a patient, the x-ray exposure is terminated. This determines the exposure time and therefore the resulting density. (See p. 232.)

RADIATION-MEASURING DEVICES

Detectors are the AEC devices that measure the amount of radiation transmitted. The radiographer selects which of the three detectors will be used. (See p. 232.)

FUNCTION OF THE IONIZATION CHAMBER

The ionization chamber interacts with transmitted radiation before it reaches the film. Air in the chamber is ionized, and an electric charge that is proportional to the amount of radiation is created. (See p. 234.)

ACCURATE PART CENTERING AND DETECTOR SELECTION

Accurate centering and detector selection are critical with AEC systems because the radiograph will demonstrate optimal density of the anatomy located directly over the detector. If the area of radiographic interest is not directly over the selected detector, that area will be overexposed or underexposed. (See p. 239.)

FUNCTION OF BACKUP TIME

Backup time, the maximum exposure time allowed during an AEC examination, serves as a safety mechanism when the AEC is not used or is not functioning properly. (See p. 241.)

SETTING BACKUP TIME

Backup time should be set at 150% to 200% of the expected exposure time. This allows the properly used AEC system to appropriately terminate the exposure but protects the patient and tube from excessive exposure if a problem occurs. (See p. 242.)

THE PATIENT AND AEC

When an AEC device is used, if the anatomic area directly over the detector does not represent the anatomic area of radiographic interest, inappropriate density may result. This can happen when the anatomic area over the detector contains a foreign object, a pocket of air, or contrast media or the anatomic area does not cover the detector completely. (See p. 242.)

Chapter 12: Computed Radiography

MATRIX SIZE AND IMAGE QUALITY

Increasing the matrix size increases the number of pixels, thereby increasing the quality of the image. Decreasing the matrix size decreases the number of pixels, thereby decreasing the quality of the image. (See p. 275.)

PIXEL NUMBER AND SPATIAL DETAIL

Increasing the number of pixels in the image matrix increases the spatial detail. (See p. 283.)

WINDOW LEVEL AND IMAGE BRIGHTNESS

A direct relationship exists between window level and image brightness on the CRT monitor. Increasing the window level increases the image brightness; decreasing the window level decreases the image brightness. (See p. 284.)

WINDOW WIDTH AND RADIOGRAPHIC CONTRAST

A narrow window (decreased) width increases radiographic contrast, whereas a wider window (increased) width decreases radiographic contrast. (p. 286.)

NUMBER OF PHOTONS AND QUANTUM MOTTLE

Decreasing the number of photons reaching the imaging plate increases the amount of quantum mottle within the image; increasing the number of photons reaching the imaging plate decreases the amount of quantum mottle within the image. (See p. 287.)

Summary of Mathematical Applications

Chapter 4: Radiographic Image Quality

ADJUSTING MILLIAMPERAGE, EXPOSURE TIME, OR BOTH TO CONTROL DENSITY

100 mA @ 0.10 s = 10 mAs. To increase the mAs to 20, you could use:

$$200 \text{ mA @ } 0.10 \text{ s} = 20 \text{ mAs}$$
$$100 \text{ mA @ } 0.20 \text{ s} = 20 \text{ mAs}$$
$$400 \text{ mA @ } 0.05 \text{ s} = 20 \text{ mAs}$$

(See p. 55.)

USING THE 15% RULE

To increase density: Multiply the kVp by 1.15 (original kVp + 15%).

$$80 \text{ kVp} \times 1.15 = 92 \text{ kVp}$$

To decrease density: Multiply the kVp by 0.85 (original kVp – 15%).

$$80 \text{ kVp} \times 0.85 = 68 \text{ kVp}$$

To maintain density:

When increasing kVp by 15% (kVp × 1.15), divide the original mAs by 2.

$$80 \text{ kVp} \times 1.15 = 92 \text{ kVp and mAs/2}$$

When decreasing the kVp by 15% (kVp × 0.85), multiply the mAs by 2.

$$80 \text{ kVp} \times 0.85 = 68 \text{ kVp and mAs} \times 2$$

(See p. 60.)

DENSITY MAINTENANCE FORMULA

$$\frac{\text{mAs}_1}{\text{mAs}_2} = \frac{(\text{SID})^2_1}{(\text{SID})^2_2}$$

For example, optimal density is achieved at an SID of 40 inches using 25 mAs. The SID must be increased to 56 inches. What adjustment in mAs is needed to maintain radiographic density?

$$\frac{25}{mAs_2} = \frac{(40)^2}{(56)^2}; \ 1600 \times = 78{,}400; \ \frac{78{,}400}{1600}; \ mAs_2 = 49$$

(See p. 61.)

ADJUSTING mAs FOR CHANGES IN PART THICKNESS

An optimal radiograph was obtained using 40 mAs on an anatomic part that measured 18 cm. The same anatomic part is radiographed in another patient, and it measures 22 cm. What new mAs is needed to maintain density? Because the part thickness was increased by 4 cm, the original mAs is multiplied by 2, yielding 80 mAs. (See p. 64.)

CALCULATING GEOMETRIC UNSHARPNESS

The amount of geometric unsharpness can be calculated for each of the following images to determine which image has increased geometric unsharpness.

Image 1
Focal spot size = 0.6 mm

SID = 40 inches

OID = 0.25 inch

Image 2
Focal spot size = 1.2 mm

SID = 56 inches

OID = 4.0 inches

Image 1
$$\frac{0.6 \text{ mm} \times 0.25 \text{ inch}}{39.75 \text{ inches}}; \frac{0.15}{39.75}$$

Image 2
$$\frac{1.2 \text{ mm} \times 4 \text{ inches}}{52 \text{ inches}}; \frac{4.8}{52}$$

Geometric unsharpness of Image 1 = 0.004 mm
Geometric unsharpness of Image 2 = 0.09 mm

Image 2 has the greatest amount of unsharpness.
(See p. 84.)

THE MAGNIFICATION FACTOR

A posteroanterior (PA) projection of the chest was produced with an SID of 72 inches and an OID of 3 inches. What is the MF?

$$MF = \frac{72 \text{ inches}}{69 \text{ inches}}$$

$$MF = 1.044$$

(See p. 92.)

DETERMINING OBJECT SIZE

On a PA chest film taken with an SID of 72 inches and an OID of 3 inches (SOD is equal to 69 inches), the size of a round lesion in the right lung measures 1.5 inches in diameter on the radiograph. The MF has been determined to be 1.044. What is the object size of this lesion?

$$\text{Object size} = \frac{1.5 \text{ inches}}{1.044}$$

$$\text{Object size} = 1.44 \text{ inches}$$

(See p. 92.)

Chapter 5: Scatter Control

USING A GRID

If a radiographer produced a knee radiograph with a nongrid exposure using 10 mAs and on the next exposure wanted to use an 8:1 grid, what mAs should be used to produce a radiograph of the same density?

Nongrid exposure = 10 mAs
8:1 grid
GCF = 4 (from Table 5-2)

$$\textbf{GCF} = \frac{\textbf{mAs with a grid}}{\textbf{mAs without the grid}}$$

$$\text{Step One: } 4 = \frac{\text{mAs}}{10}$$

$$\text{Step Two: } (4)(10) = \text{mAs}$$

$$\text{Step Three: } 40 = \text{mAs with a grid}$$

NOTE: mAs must be increased by a factor of 4 to 40 mAs.
(See p. 120.)

NOT USING A GRID

If a radiographer produced a knee radiograph using a 16:1 grid and 60 mAs and on the next exposure wanted to use a nongrid exposure, what mAs should be used to produce a radiograph of the same density?

Grid exposure = 60 mAs
16:1 grid
GCF = 6 (from Table 5-2)

$$\textbf{GCF} = \frac{\textbf{mAs with a grid}}{\textbf{mAs without the grid}}$$

$$\text{Step One: } 6 = \frac{60}{\text{mAs}}$$

$$\text{Step Two: } (\text{mAs})(6) = \left(\frac{60}{\text{mAs}}\right)(\text{mAs})$$

$$\text{Step Three: } \text{mAs} = (60)\left(\frac{1}{6}\right)$$

$$\text{Step Four: } \text{mAs} = 10$$

NOTE: mAs must be decreased by a factor of 6 to 10 mAs.
(See pp. 120-121.)

INCREASING THE GRID RATIO

If a radiographer performed a routine portable kidney, ureter, and bladder (KUB) examination using 30 mAs with a 6:1 grid, what mAs should be used if a 12:1 grid were used?

30 mAs, 6:1 grid, Bucky factor = 3

_____ mAs, 12:1 grid, Bucky factor = 5

$$\frac{\text{mAs}_1}{\text{mAs}_2} = \frac{\text{BF}_1}{\text{BF}_2}$$

$$\text{Step One: } \frac{30}{\text{mAs}_2} = \frac{3}{5}$$

Step Two: Simply cross multiply:
$$(\text{mAs}_2)(3) = (30)(5)$$

$$\text{Step Three: } \text{mAs}_2 = \frac{(30)(5)}{3}$$

$$\text{Step Four: } \text{mAs}_2 = 50 \text{ mAs}$$

(See p. 121.)

DECREASING THE GRID RATIO

If a radiographer used 37.5 mAs with an 8:1 grid, what mAs should be used with a 5:1 grid?

37.5 mAs, 8:1 grid, Bucky factor = 4

_____ mAs, 5:1 grid, Bucky factor = 2

$$\frac{\text{mAs}_1}{\text{mAs}_2} = \frac{\text{BF}_1}{\text{BF}_2}$$

$$\text{Step One: } \frac{37.5}{\text{mAs}_2} = \frac{4}{2}$$

$$\text{Step Two: } (mAs_2)(4) = (37.5)(2)$$

$$\text{Step Three: } mAs_2 = \frac{(37.5)(2)}{4}$$

$$\text{Step Four: } mAs_2 = 18.75 \text{ mAs}$$

(See p. 122.)

Chapter 6: Image Receptors

THE INTENSIFICATION FACTOR

If a radiograph of a hand was produced with 100 mAs using direct exposure and a radiograph of the same hand was produced with an intensifying screen system using 4 mAs, resulting in the same density as the first film, what is the IF of the screen system?

$$IF = \frac{100 \text{ mAs}}{4 \text{ mAs}}$$

$$IF = 25$$

This indicates that 25 times the exposure would be needed to produce a radiograph with comparable density if a direct-exposure system was used. (See p. 148.)

USE OF THE mAs CONVERSION FORMULA FOR SCREENS

If 10 mAs were used with a 400 speed screen system to produce an optimal radiograph, what mAs would be necessary to produce a radiograph with the same density using a 100 speed screen system?

$$\frac{10 \text{ mAs}}{mAs_2} = \frac{100 \text{ relative speed}}{400 \text{ relative speed}}$$

$$mAs_2 = 40$$

(See p. 149.)

Chapter 8: Sensitometry

USING SENSITOMETRY TO CALCULATE EXPOSURE TECHNIQUE CHANGES

60 mAs produced an image density of 2.05 (log E = 1.54). What mAs would produce an image density of 1.30 (log E = 1.38)?

Subtract log E of the original density (2.05) from the log E of the desired density (1.30):

$$\begin{array}{r} 1.38 \\ -\ 1.54 \\ \hline -\ 0.16; \text{ antilog of } -0.16 = 0.69 \end{array}$$

Multiply the original mAs by 0.69:

$$60 \text{ mAs} \times 0.69 = 41.4 \text{ mAs}$$

Changing the original optical density on the repeat radiograph from 2.05 to 1.30 requires that the mAs needs be decreased to 41.4. (See p. 205.)

CALCULATING AVERAGE GRADIENT

$$\text{Average gradient} = \frac{D_2 - D_1}{E_2 - E_1}$$

where

$$D_1 = \text{OD } 0.25 + 0.17 \text{ (B + F)}$$
$$D_2 = \text{OD } 2.0 + 0.17 \text{ (B + F)}$$
$$E_1 = \text{Exposure that produces } D_1$$
$$E_2 = \text{Exposure that produces } D_2$$

Example:

$$\frac{2.17 - 0.42}{1.46 - 0.8} = 1.75 = 2.65 \text{ Average gradient } 0.66$$

(See p. 207.)

Summary of Practical Tips

Chapter 3: Radiographic Image Formation

X-Ray Interaction with Matter

When the primary x-ray beam interacts with anatomic tissues, three processes occur during attenuation of the x-ray beam: absorption, scattering, and transmission. (See p. 46.)

Chapter 4: Radiographic Image Quality

Repeating Radiographs Because of Density Errors

The minimum change needed to correct for a density error is determined by multiplying or dividing the mAs by 2. When a greater change in mAs is needed, the radiographer should multiply or divide by 4, 8, and so on. (See p. 57.)

Kilovoltage and the 15% Rule

A 15% increase in kilovoltage peak will have the same effect on radiographic density as doubling the mAs. A 15% decrease in kVp will have the same effect on radiographic density as decreasing the mAs by half. (See p. 59.)

Altering SID between 40 and 72 Inches

When a 72-inch SID cannot be used, adjusting the SID to 56 inches requires half the mAs. When a 40-inch SID cannot be used, adjusting the SID to 56 inches requires twice the mAs. This quick method of calculating mAs changes should produce sufficient density. (See p. 61.)

Selecting Focal Spot Size

The radiographer should select the smallest focal spot size, considering the amount of x-ray exposure used and the amount of recorded detail required for the radiographic examination. (See p. 80.)

MINIMIZING GEOMETRIC UNSHARPNESS

The radiographer should select the smallest focal spot size when maximal recorded detail is important; he or she should also consider the amount of heat load within the x-ray tube. In addition, the radiographer should select the standard SID when OID is minimal. When increased OID is unavoidable, the SID should be increased slightly to compensate. (See p. 84.)

ELIMINATING MOTION

Patient motion can be controlled by the radiographer by doing the following:

1. Using short exposure times compensated for by higher mA
2. Communicating good instructions for the patient to assist in immobilization
3. Using physical immobilization, such as sandbags, tape, or other devices, as deemed necessary

If a patient needs to be physically held, it is generally recommended that the holder not be a person who routinely is exposed to x-rays. The holder should always wear lead shielding and, if female, be evaluated for the possibility of pregnancy before making the exposure. (See p. 88.)

MINIMIZING OID

The radiographer should always try to minimize OID as much as possible to reduce size distortion (magnification). Within the protocol of the examination, it is always best to try to position the area of interest closest to the image receptor to minimize size distortion of that area. (See p. 90.)

MINIMIZING SHAPE DISTORTION

Elongation and foreshortening can be minimized by ensuring the proper CR alignment of the following:

1. X-ray tube
2. Part
3. Image receptor
4. Entry or exit point of the CR

(See p. 94.)

Chapter 5: Scatter Control

COMPENSATING FOR COLLIMATION

When collimating significantly (changing from a 11×14 inch field size to a small, 4-inch-diameter cone), the radiographer must increase exposure to compensate for the loss of density that will otherwise occur. The kilovoltage peak (kVp) value should not be increased. Increasing the kVp value will decrease contrast. To change density only, the product of milliamperage and exposure time (mAs) should be changed. (See p. 105.)

LIMITING FIELD SIZE TO IMAGE RECEPTOR SIZE

The size of the projected radiation field should never exceed the size of the image receptor. This will ensure patient protection from excessive radiation exposure while also improving image quality. (See p. 111.)

GRID SELECTION

Grids differ from one another in performance, especially regarding grid ratio and focal distance. Before using a grid, the radiographer must determine the grid ratio so that the appropriate exposure factors can be selected. Also, the radiographer must be aware of the focal range of focused grids, or the minimum SID of parallel grids, so that the appropriate SID is selected. In addition, if the grid is mounted to a cassette, the film-screen speed should be determined before the exposure factors are selected. (See p. 118.)

OID AND THE AIR GAP TECHNIQUE

Using an increased OID is a necessity for the air gap technique. However, this decreases image quality. To decrease magnification and increase recorded detail when using the air gap technique, the radiographer must increase SID. (See p. 130.)

Chapter 6: Image Receptors

SPECTRAL EMISSION AND SPECTRAL SENSITIVITY

The spectral emission of intensifying screens must be matched to the spectral sensitivity of the film. It is also important to make sure that the spectral emission of safelight filters in the darkroom is compatible with the spectral sensitivity of the film. (See p. 143.)

SELECTING A SCREEN SPEED

The radiographer should select the film-screen system that will balance patient exposure and recorded detail. (See p. 150.)

IDENTIFYING CASSETTES

When it is necessary to find the specific cassette that has a problem, it can be done easily by numbering the cassettes. An excellent way to accomplish this is to write the cassette number (using a permanent black marker) on the surface of one of the screens in a corner out of the way. That same number then needs to be written on the outside of the cassette. The screen number will show up on images produced with that cassette, and if there is a problem, knowing this number will allow the radiographer to find and test the cassette in question. (See p. 154.)

Chapter 7: Radiographic Processing

FILM ORIENTATION FOR PROPER REPLENISHMENT

The radiographer should align the radiographic film so that the film is horizontally placed on the feedtray and its leading edge is long. When processing two 8×10 inch films, the radiographer should place both films parallel to each other so that the leading edges are short. (See p. 175.)

Chapter 8: Sensitometry

SENSITOMETRIC CURVES POSITION ALONG THE X AXIS

Sensitometric curves of faster-speed film are positioned to the left of slower-speed film, and sensitometric curves of slower-speed film are positioned to the right of faster-speed film. (See p. 203.)

CHANGES IN EXPOSURE TECHNIQUE TO CORRECT FOR DENSITY ERRORS

Optical densities that lie outside the straight-line region of the sensitometric curve (toe or shoulder region) require a greater or lesser proportional change than those that lie within the straight-line region to correct for the density error. (See p. 210.)

ACHIEVING MAXIMUM FILM CONTRAST

To achieve the maximum contrast the film is capable of producing, the radiographer must ensure that the optical densities lie within the straight-line region of the sensitometric curve. (See p. 211.)

Chapter 9: Exposure Factor Selection

TECHNIQUE CHART LIMITATIONS

Exposure technique charts are designed for the typical or average patient. Patient variability in terms of body habitus, physical condition, or the presence of a pathologic condition requires the radiographer to problem solve when selecting exposure factors. (See p. 217.)

EQUIPMENT PERFORMANCE

Radiographic equipment must be operating within normal limits for technique charts to be effective. (See p. 218.)

MEASUREMENT OF PART THICKNESS

Accurate measurement of part thickness is critical to the effective use of exposure technique charts. (See p. 218.)

APPLICABILITY OF A VARIABLE kVp/FIXED mAs TECHNIQUE CHART

Variable kVp technique charts may be more effective when small extremities are being imaged. (See p. 221.)

FIXED kVp/VARIABLE mAs AND PART MEASUREMENT

Accuracy of measurement is less critical with fixed kVp/variable mAs technique charts than with variable kVp/fixed mAs technique charts. (See p. 223.)

Chapter 10: Automatic Exposure Controls

FILM-SCREEN SYSTEMS AND AEC

When an AEC system is used, the radiographer must be certain to use the film-screen system for which the AEC system was calibrated. If more than one film-screen system is used in a department, the radiographer should use the system for which the AEC system was calibrated. (See p. 235.)

PATIENT MOTION AND AEC

Because the minimum response time for AEC is longer than for other types of radiographic timers, the radiographer must decide carefully whether the AEC should be used for particular patients and examinations. If a patient is unable to cooperate in remaining still or holding his or her breath, the use of an AEC device probably is not the best choice. The radiographer should instead set a manual technique rather than use the AEC to prevent the imaging of patient motion. (See p. 235.)

CALIBRATION AND UNACCEPTABLE RADIOGRAPHS

If radiographs produced in a specific room using an AEC device consistently have too much or too little density, the radiographer should be sure to check the calibration of the AEC system (or have it checked). (See p. 236.)

AEC, kVp, AND RADIOGRAPHIC CONTRAST

Assuming the radiographer is selecting or using a kVp value above the minimum needed to penetrate the part, adjusting this value will not affect density when using an AEC device. It will affect radiographic contrast, however (Figure 10-7). The radiographer must be sure to set the kVp value as needed to ensure adequate penetration and to produce the appropriate scale of contrast. (See p. 239.)

AEC AND DENSITY SETTINGS

Routinely using plus or minus density settings to produce acceptable radiographs indicates that a problem exists, possibly a problem with the AEC device. (See p. 240.)

AEC AND NON-BUCKY STUDIES

The radiographer should be certain to deactivate the AEC system and use manual technique when doing any radiographic study where the film is located outside of the Bucky. (See p. 243.)

AEC AND mAs READOUT

If the radiographic unit has a mAs readout display, the radiographer should be sure to notice what it reads after the exposure is made. This information can be invaluable. (See p. 244.)

Chapter 11: Exposure Factor Modification

PEDIATRIC CHEST EXPOSURE TIME

An exposure time of 0.0083 s ($\frac{1}{120}$ s) should be used to minimize the appearance of motion on the radiograph. (See p. 250.)

PEDIATRIC SKULL RADIOGRAPHY

The radiographer should decrease the kVp value by 15% from an adult technique for skull radiography when performed on pediatric patients younger than 6 years old. (See p. 251.)

EXPOSURE MODIFICATION FOR CHANGES IN PATIENT POSITION FROM AP TO LATERAL/OBLIQUE POSITIONS

The radiographer should increase the kVp value by 15% (2 × mAs) for each additional centimeter of tissue caused by moving the patient from an AP position to a lateral or oblique position. This increase in kVp will maintain density for the oblique and lateral radiographs. (See p. 254.)

EXPOSURE MODIFICATION FOR LATERAL LUMBAR SPINE RADIOGRAPHS

Part thickness should not be measured through the central ray. The radiographer should measure the AP projection just below the tip of the sternum and the lateral projection at the level of L2. As previously discussed, the kVp value should be increased by 15% (2 × mAs) for each additional centimeter of tissue caused by moving the patient from an AP position to a lateral position. (See p. 255.)

EXPOSURE FACTOR SELECTION FOR FIBERGLASS CASTING MATERIALS

Fiberglass casts require no change in exposure factors from the usual technique for that body part. (See p. 255.)

EXPOSURE FACTOR SELECTION FOR PLASTER CASTING MATERIALS

Plaster casts require at least 2 times the mAs (or an increased kVp value by 15%) from the usual technique, but they may require more based on the thickness of the casting material. (See p. 256.)

EXPOSURE FACTOR SELECTION FOR SPLINTS

If an aluminum, wood, or solid plastic splint is located in the path of the primary beam, mAs must be increased by 50% to produce a quality radiograph. (See p. 256.)

CHANGING kVp TO COMPENSATE FOR PATHOLOGIC CONDITIONS

The radiographer should adjust kVp by at least 15% when compensating for pathologic conditions. (See p. 262.)

CHANGING EXPOSURE FACTORS TO VISUALIZE SOFT TISSUE

The radiographer should decrease kVp by 15% from the usual technique of the same body part when a soft tissue examination is warranted. (See p. 263.)

SELECTION OF EXPOSURE FACTORS FOR USE WITH CONTRAST MEDIA

The radiographer should select a high kVp (90 and above) for barium sulfate studies and a medium kVp (70 to 80) for procedures requiring iodinated solutions. (See p. 264.)

COMPENSATING EXPOSURE FACTORS FOR CHANGING GENERATOR TYPE

To maintain radiographic density and contrast, the radiographer must decrease the kVp value by 15% for three-phase generators and high-frequency generators compared with single-phase generators. (See p. 266.)

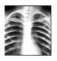

Film Critique Interpretations

Chapter 4: Radiographic Image Quality

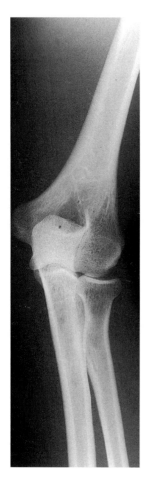
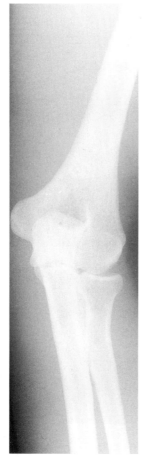
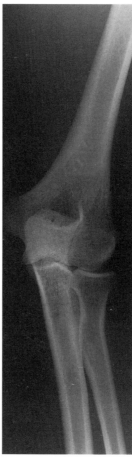
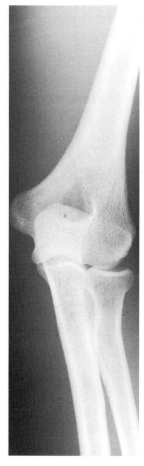

FIGURE 4-34 Image A was produced using 60 kVp, 100 mA at 0.040 s, 100 speed film-screen combination, 40-inch SID, and minimal OID.

FIGURE 4-35 Image B was produced using 60 kVp, 80 mA at 0.025 s, 100 speed film-screen combination, 40-inch SID, and minimal OID.

FIGURE 4-36 Image C was produced using 69 kVp, 160 mA at 0.025 s, 100 speed film-screen combination, 40-inch SID, and minimal OID.

FIGURE 4-37 Image D was produced using 60 kVp, 200 mA at 0.020 s, 100 speed film-screen combination, 40-inch SID, and 3-inch OID.

1. Given Image A is of optimal quality, discuss the quality of the other images.

   Image B The radiographic density of this image is insufficient (too light) to visualize all of the anatomic structures. Radiographic contrast and recorded detail cannot be evaluated because the image is too light.

   Image C The radiographic density of this image is too excessive (too dark) to adequately visualize all of the anatomic structures. Radiographic contrast and recorded detail cannot be evaluated because the image is too dark.

   Image D The radiographic density of this image is slightly lower than that in Image A. Radiographic contrast appears slightly higher than that of Image A. Differences in recorded detail are difficult to visualize, but the image appears magnified in comparison to Image A.

2. For each image, evaluate its exposure variables and discuss their effect on the quality of the image, regardless of whether it is apparent on the radiograph.

   Image B The kVp is the same as that used in Image A; therefore the radiographic contrast would be equal. The mAs used is 2, demonstrating a change from Image A by half, resulting in the radiographic density being half as dark. All other exposure factors remain the same, producing the same amount of recorded detail as in Image A.

   Image C The kVp is 15% higher than the kVp used in Image A. This increases the density by a factor of 2. The mAs used (4) is the same as used in Image A (4). All other exposure factors are equal, so the amount of recorded detail is equal to that of Image A.

   Image D The kVp and mAs are the same as those used in Image A. The only exposure factor changed is the object-to-image receptor distance (OID). An increase in OID (3 inches) increases the size of the image (magnification) and results in less scatter radiation reaching the film. This increases the radiographic contrast and decreases radiographic density.

3. For each image, identify any adjustments that could be made in the exposure factors to produce an image comparable to Image A.

   Image B To increase the radiographic density by a factor of 2, the radiographer must increase the mAs by a factor of 2. The mA can be doubled (160 mA at 0.025 = 4 mAs), or the time of exposure can be doubled (80 mA at 0.050 = 4 mAs).

   Image C To decrease the radiographic density, the radiographer must decrease the mAs by a factor of 2 or decrease the kVp by 15%. A kVp of 69 produces lower radiographic contrast than a kVp of 60. Therefore changing the kVp to 60 (a 15% decrease) will decrease the radiographic density by half and produce an image comparable to Image A.

   Image D Maintaining the same exposure factors and decreasing the OID to minimal will produce an image comparable to Image A. Decreasing the OID will produce an image with less magnification and add slightly more density because more scatter radiation will reach the film.

Chapter 5: Scatter Control

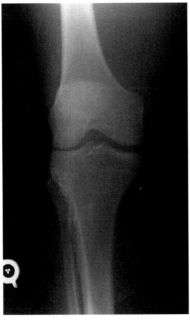 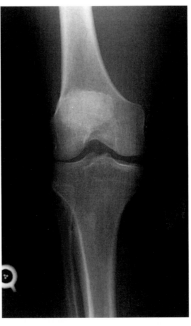

FIGURE 5-28 Image A was produced using 70 kVp, 100 mA at 0.016 s, 400 speed film-screen combination, a 40-inch source-to-image receptor distance, and no grid.

FIGURE 5-29 Image B was produced using 70 kVp, 50 mA at 0.160 s, 400 speed film-screen combination, a 40-inch source-to-image receptor distance, and a 12:1 grid ratio.

1. Evaluate each radiograph and discuss its quality.

   Image A The radiographic density is sufficient to visualize the anatomic structures. Radiographic contrast appears low, decreasing the visibility of recorded detail. The recorded detail is difficult to evaluate, but unsharpness appears minimal.

   Image B The radiographic density is sufficient to visualize the anatomic structures. The radiographic contrast appears high, and visibility of recorded detail is improved compared with that of Image A. The recorded detail is difficult to evaluate, but unsharpness appears minimal.

2. For each image, evaluate its exposure variables and discuss their effect on the quality of the image, regardless of whether it is apparent on the radiograph.

   Image A This image was produced using a nongrid exposure technique. A nongrid exposure technique on an adult knee will produce an image with lower radiographic contrast because more scatter radiation reaches the film. The kVp used (70) is the same as that used in Image B. The mAs is less to compensate for the nongrid exposure. The density and recorded detail should be similar to those of Image B.

Image B This image was produced using a 12:1 grid ratio. The result is a higher-contrast image because less scatter radiation reaches the film. The mAs was increased to compensate for the use of a grid. The density and recorded detail should be similar to those of Image A.

3. For each image, identify any adjustments that could be made in the exposure factors to produce an optimal image?

Image A To increase the radiographic contrast and improve the quality of the image, the radiographer can add a 12:1 grid. The mAs would need to be increased by a factor of 5 to compensate for adding the grid. The new mAs would be 8.

Image B No adjustments need to be made to improve the quality of this image.

Chapter 6: Image Receptors

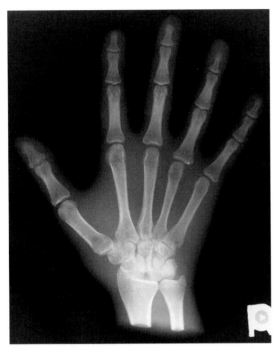

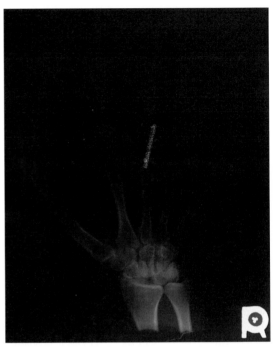

FIGURE 6-16 Image A was produced using 57 kVp, 50 mA at 0.040 s, 100 speed film-screen combination, and a 40-inch source-to-image receptor distance.

FIGURE 6-17 Image B was produced using 57 kVp, 160 mA at 0.0125 s, 400 speed film-screen combination, and a 40-inch source-to-image receptor distance.

1. Evaluate each radiograph and discuss its quality.

   Image A The radiographic density is sufficient to visualize the anatomic structures. The radiographic contrast is appropriate to visualize the recorded detail. The recorded detail is difficult to evaluate, but unsharpness appears minimal.

   Image B The radiographic density is excessive (too dark), thereby decreasing the visualization of the anatomic structures. The radiographic contrast and recorded detail cannot be evaluated.

2. For each image, evaluate its exposure variables and discuss their effect on the quality of the image, regardless of whether it is apparent on the radiograph.

   Image A The kVp (57) used is appropriate for the level of contrast desired for an extremity radiograph. The mAs (2) used produced sufficient density to visualize the anatomic structures. A 100 film-screen speed combination is appropriate to provide maximum recorded detail.

   Image B The kVp (57) used is appropriate for the level of contrast desired for an extremity radiograph. The mAs (2) used is appropriate for a slower film-screen speed combination. The 400 speed film-screen combination used produced an image with 4 times the density compared with that of Image A. In addition, the recorded detail is lower because of the higher screen speed.

3. For each image, identify any adjustments that could be made in the exposure factors to produce an optimal image?

Image A No adjustments need to be made to improve the quality of this image.

Image B The kVp and mAs are adequate for producing a quality image of the hand. The 400 speed film-screen combination should be changed to a 100 speed film-screen combination. This would decrease the radiographic density by a factor of 4. In the event that a lower speed film-screen combination could not be used, the mAs needs to be decreased by a factor of 4 to decrease the radiographic density. The new mAs used with the 400 speed film-screen combination would be 0.5.

Chapter 10: AEC

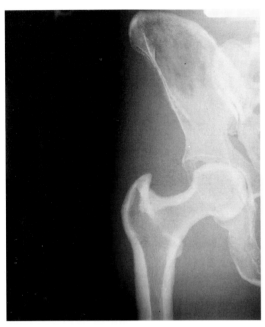

FIGURE 10-9 Image A was produced using 70 kVp, 200 mA, AEC exposure, center detector, 400 speed film-screen combination, and a 40-inch source-to-image receptor distance.

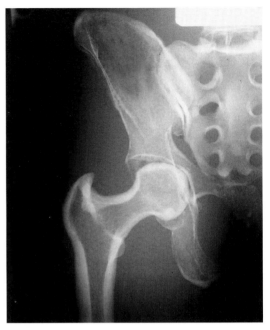

FIGURE 10-10 Image B was produced using 70 kVp, 200 mA, AEC exposure, center detector, 400 speed film-screen combination, and a 40-inch source-to-image receptor distance.

1. Evaluate each radiograph and discuss its quality.

   Image A The radiographic density is low, thereby reducing the visibility of some anatomic structures. The radiographic contrast appears appropriate for the anatomic structure. The recorded detail is difficult to evaluate, but unsharpness appears minimal. The central ray centering appears more lateral compared with the positioning used in Image B.

   Image B The radiographic density is sufficient to visualize the anatomic structure. The radiographic contrast is appropriate to visualize the recorded detail. The recorded detail is difficult to evaluate, but unsharpness appears minimal. The central ray centering appears more medial compared with the positioning used in Image A.

2. For each image, evaluate its exposure variables and discuss their effect on the quality of the image, regardless of whether it is apparent on the radiograph.

   Image A The kVp is appropriate for the anatomic structure. The film-screen combination and AEC center detector are appropriate for the hip. The exposure factors are the same as those used in Image B. Although image quality is not equal, exposure factors appear appropriate for the examination.

Image B The kVp is appropriate for the anatomic structure. The film-screen combination and AEC center detector are appropriate for the hip. The exposure factors are the same as those used in Image A. Although image quality is not equal, exposure factors appear appropriate for the examination.

3. For each image, identify any adjustments that could be made in the exposure factors to produce an optimal image.

Image A Given an AEC exposure and the same factors used in Image B, the centering of the central ray needs to be directed more medially and centered closer to the femoral neck. Improper centering of the central ray produced an image with less density because the hip was not placed correctly over the center detector.

Image B No adjustments need to be made to improve the quality of this image.

Answer Key

Chapter 1: Radiation and Its Discovery

1. B
2. C
3. D
4. A
5. D
6. C
7. B
8. D
9. A
10. C

Chapter 2: Production of X-Rays

1. B
2. D
3. B
4. A
5. C
6. A
7. D
8. A
9. C
10. D

Chapter 3: Radiographic Image Formation

1. D
2. D
3. C
4. B
5. D

6. B
7. A
8. C
9. C
10. A

Chapter 4: Radiographic Image Quality

1. B
2. D
3. C
4. D
5. A
6. B
7. B
8. B
9. A
10. C
11. B
12. C
13. B
14. D
15. D
16. A
17. B
18. C
19. D
20. A

Chapter 5: Scatter Control

1. C
2. A
3. D
4. B
5. B
6. A
7. D
8. D
9. B
10. A

11. D
12. B
13. C
14. C
15. A
16. B
17. C
18. D

Chapter 6: Image Receptors

1. A
2. C
3. A
4. B
5. C
6. C
7. C
8. D
9. B
10. D
11. B
12. C
13. A
14. C
15. D

Chapter 7: Radiographic Processing

1. B
2. C
3. C
4. A
5. D
6. C
7. B
8. C
9. D
10. A
11. C
12. D

13. C
14. B
15. A

Chapter 8: Sensitometry

1. D
2. B
3. D
4. B
5. A
6. C
7. B
8. A
9. A
10. D

Chapter 9: Exposure Factor Selection

1. C
2. B
3. C
4. A
5. D
6. B
7. C
8. B
9. D
10. A

Chapter 10: Automatic Exposure Control

1. C
2. B
3. C
4. D
5. D
6. B
7. D

8. B
9. A
10. C

Chapter 11: Exposure Factor Modification

1. C
2. B
3. A
4. C
5. D
6. C
7. D

Chapter 12: Computed Radiography

1. B
2. D
3. B
4. D
5. B
6. C
7. C
8. C
9. A
10. B

INDEX

A

Abdomen, radiograph of, *75*, 264
Absorbing layer of intensifying screen, 146
Absorption
    beam attenuation and, 43-44, *44*
    differential, *42*, 42-48
Absorption efficiency, screen speed and, 150
Accelerator agent, developing and, 165
Accurate part centering and detector selection, 239
Acetic acid, 167, 168*t*
Acid, 167
Acidifier, fixing and, 167
Activator agent, developing and, 165
Active layer of intensifying screen, 146
Actual focal spot size, 31
ADC; *see* Analog-to-digital converter
Added filtration, 33, *34*
Adhesive, radiographic film and, 138
AEC; *see* Automatic exposure control
AEDs; *see* Automatic exposure devices
Aerial oxidation, 173
Afterglow, 145
Ag; *see* Silver
AgBr; *see* Silver bromide
AgI; *see* Silver iodide
Air gap technique
    object-to-image receptor distance and, 130
    scatter control and, 129-131, *130*, 131*t*
Algorithms, 277-278
Aluminum, millimeters of, 34
Aluminum-added filtration, *34*
Aluminum chloride, 167, 168*t*
Aluminum salt, 167
Aluminum sulfate, 167, 168*t*
Ammonium thiosulfate, 166, 167, 168*t*
Analog-to-digital converter (ADC), 270-271
Anatomic part
    radiographic contrast and, *74*, *75*, 75-76
    radiographic density and, 64-65

Anatomic programming, automatic exposure control and, *244*, 244-245
Anatomically programmed radiography (APR), 244, *244*, *245*
Anatomy, comparative, exposure technique charts and, 224
Angstroms, 6
Ankle radiograph, *253*
Anode, 14, 25, 38
    rotating, 17-18
    x-ray production and, 15-18, *16*, *17*
Anode heel effect, 31-32, *33*, 65
Anteroposterior (AP) radiograph, 65, 243, 251-253, *252*, *253*, 254, *254*
Anticurl/antihalation layer, screen film and, 140-141
Antilog, 205
AP radiograph; *see* Anteroposterior radiograph
Aperture diaphragms, beam restriction and, 106, *106*, *107*
APR; *see* Anatomically programmed radiography
Archival quality of radiographs, 168, 169, 180
Artifacts, radiographic, 185, 186*t*-187*t*, 188*t*-189*t*
Asthenic type of body habitus, 257-259
Asymmetric screens, 144
Attentuation, beam, 43-48
Automatic collimators, beam restriction and, 111
Automatic exposure control (AEC), 216, 228-247, 250
    anatomic programming and, 244-245
    limitations of systems of, 234-236
    purpose of, 230-232
    systems of, 232-234
    technical considerations with, 236-244
Automatic exposure devices (AEDs), 230-231, 287
Automatic processing equipment, 162, *164*
Automatic processor, 162, *164*
    cross-section of, *170*
    tanks of, 169
Average gradient, *206*, 207-208

Page numbers in *italics* indicate illustrations; *t* indicates tables.

B

B + F; *see* Base plus fog

Back screen of intensifying screen, 146

Backup time
  automatic exposure control and, 241-242
  function of, 241
  setting, 242

Barium fluorohalide crystals, 275

Barium platinocyanide, 3

Base
  of intensifying screen, 146
  plus fog (B + F), 198

Base layer, radiographic film and, 137

Beam, x-ray; *see* X-ray beam

Beam filtration, 32-35, *34*

Beam penetrability, x-ray quality and, 28

Beam restriction, 103-105, *104*, 109

Beam-restricting devices, 102
  scatter control and, *102*, 102-103
  types of, 105-111

Black/white reversal, computed radiography
  and, 278

Blue-sensitive film, 141-142

Blur, 87

Body habitus, exposure factor modification and,
  257-258, 257-259

Br; *see* Bromide

Bremsstrahlung interactions, 20, *21*

Bromide (Br), 138, 165

Bucky, Gustave, 112

Bucky factor, 119, 120, 121

Bucky selection, automatic exposure control and,
  243

Buffer, 167

Buffering agent, 165

C

Calcium tungstate, 147, 151

Calculator, exposure technique charts and, 223-224

Calibration, lack of, automatic exposure control
  and, 236

Calipers
  exposure technique charts and, 223-224
  in measurement of part thickness, 218, *219*

Camera, laser, printing and, computed radiography
  and, 282

Carbonate, buffering agent and, 165

Cassettes, 155-157, *156*
  filmless, 272
  grid, 118
  identifying, 154

Casts
  exposure factor modification and, 255-256
  Fiberglass, exposure factor selection
    for, 255

Cathode, 14, *15*, 25

Cathode-ray-tube (CRT), 273, 278-282, *279*, *280*,
  281, 283, 284

Cells, automatic exposure control and, 232

Centering of the part, automatic exposure control
  and, 236, *237*

Cervical spine radiograph, *130*

Chamber
  automatic exposure control and, 232
  ionization; *see* Ionization chamber

Characteristic interactions, 20-21, *22*

Charts
  exposure technique, 216-219, *219*
  tube rating, 36, *37*

Chemical exposure, darkrooms and, 184

Chemical fog, restrainer and, 165

Chemicals, fixer, solvent and, 167

Chest radiograph, *71*, *72*, *74*, 237, *238*, *261*, *262*
  pediatric, exposure time for, 250, 251

Children, exposure factor modification and,
  250-251, 250*t*, 251*t*

Chrome alum, 167, 168*t*

Circular grid, 119

Classic scattering, 45

Coherent scattering, 45

Cold-water processors, 179

Collimation, 103, 105, 109
  automatic exposure control and, 241
  beam restriction and, 104-105, 105*t*
  compensating for, 105
  patient dose and, 103
  radiographic contrast and, 73, 104
  radiographic density and, 64, 105
  scatter radiation and, 104

Collimators
  automatic, 111
  beam restriction and, 109-111, *110*

Communication networks, digital, computed radiography and, 288
Comparative anatomy, exposure technique charts and, 224
Compensating exposure factors for changing generator type, 266
Compensating filter, 35
Compton effect, 44, *45*
Compton electron, 44
Computed radiography, 268-289
    characteristics of images by, *273*, 273-275, *274*
    versus conventional radiography, 271-273, *272*
    digital communication networks and, 288
    digital fluoroscopy, 270-271
    digital image quality and, 282
    direct radiography and, 287-288
    image acquisition and, 275, 276, 277
    image characteristics of, 273-275
    image display and, 278-282
    image processing and, 275-282, *278*
    limitations of conventional radiography, 271
    resolution and, 282-287
Computed tomography (CT), 270
Cones, beam restriction and, 106-109, *107*, *108*, *109*
Contrast
    beam restriction and, 104
    computed radiography and, *285*, 285-286, *286*
    film; *see* Film contrast
    maximum film, 211-212, *212*
    radiographic; *see* Radiographic contrast
Contrast agent; *see* Contrast media
Contrast enhancement, computed radiography and, 278, *280*, *281*
Contrast media
    exposure factor modification and, 263-264, *264*
    negative, 77, *77*, 264
    positive, *76*, 76-77, 263-264
    radiographic contrast and, *76*, 76-78, *77*
Conventional radiography; *see* Radiography, conventional
Convergent line, 116, *117*
Convergent point, 116, *117*
Conversion efficiency, screen speed and, 150
Crookes tube, 3, *3*
Crossed grids, *114*, 115

Cross-hatched grids, *114*, 115
Crossover
    radiographic film and, *143*, 143-144
    recorded detail and, 144
Crossover roller, 171, *172*
CRT; *see* Cathode-ray-tube
Crystal size, screen speed and, 151
Crystals, unexposed, clearing, 167
CT; *see* Computed tomography
Current
    filament, 23
    tube; *see* Tube current
Cylinders, beam restriction and, 106-109, *107*, *108*, *109*

D
Darkroom, 183-184
Deadman switches, x-ray exposure and, 23
Deep rollers, 171
Densitometer, 196, *196*
Density
    computed radiography and, *283*, 283-284, *284*
    image, 46
    optical; *see* Optical density
    radiographic, 165
    step-wedge, 195, *195*
Density errors, changes in exposure technique to correct for, 210
Density maintenance formula, 61
Density selections, automatic exposure control and, 240
Density settings, automatic exposure control and, 240
Design characteristics, exposure technique charts and, 218-219
Detector selection
    accurate part centering and, 239
    automatic exposure control and, 236-239, *238*
Detectors, automatic exposure control and, 232
Developer tank, 169
Developer temperature, radiographic quality and, 178, *180*
Developing, radiographic processing and, 163-166
Developing agents, 164-165
Diagnostic range, optical density and, 199
Differential absorption, 42-48

Diffusion, 168
Digital communication networks, computed radiography and, 288
Digital fluoroscopy, *270*, 270-271
Digital image quality, computed radiography and, 282
Digital imaging, 270
Direct radiography, computed radiography and, 287-288
Direct-exposure film, 140
Dissipating heat, anode and, 16-17
Distance
  radiographic density and, 60-61
  radiographic image quality and, *81*, 81-84, *82*, *83*
Distance decentering grid cutoff, 125-126, *127*
Distortion
  radiographic image quality and, 88-96
  size, 88-93
Double-emulsion film, 136, 140, *140*
Double-filament cathode, 14
Drying, 168-169
Drying system, radiographic processing and, 180-181, *181*
Dual nature of x-ray energy, 6
Dual-focus tubes, 14
Duplitized screen film, 140

E

Edge enhancement, computed radiography and, 278, *281*
Effective focal spot size, 31
Electrolytic silver recovery, 185
Electromagnetic radiation, 2, 6
Electromagnetic spectrum, 7
Electron volts (eV), 8
Electrons, 14
  quantity of, 30
  speed of, kilovoltage and, 28
Elongation, 93, *93*
Emission
  light, screen speed and, 148
  spectral, 142, 143
  thermionic, 23, 24
Emulsion layer, radiographic film and, 136
Energy
  properties of, 9-10
  x-rays as, 6-9, *7*, *8*

Energy conversion in x-ray tube, 26
Entrance roller assembly, 169, *170*
Equipment
  radiographic, performance of, 218
  for sensitometry, *194*, 194-196, *195*
Errors, density, changes in exposure technique to correct for, 210
Europium, computed radiography and, 275
eV; *see* Electron volts
Exit radiation, beam attenuation and, 46-48, *47*
Exposure button, x-ray exposure and, 23, *27*
Exposure control, automatic; *see* Automatic exposure control
Exposure factor modification, 248-267
  body habitus and, 257-259
  casts and splints and, 255-256
  contrast media and, 263-264
  generator type and, 265-266
  pathologic conditions and, 259-262
  for pediatric patients, 250-251
  projections and positions, 251-255
  soft tissue technique and, 262-263
Exposure factor selection, 214-227
  exposure technique chart development, 223-226
  exposure technique charts, 216-219
  for Fiberglass casting materials, 255
  for plaster casts, 255, 256
  for splints, 256
  types of technique charts, 219-223
Exposure factors, compensating, for changing generator type, 266
Exposure latitude, 141, *142*, *208*, 208-210, *209*
  film contrast and, 209
Exposure technique, changes in, to correct for density errors, 210
Exposure technique charts, 216-219, *219*, *225*
  development of, 223-226
  types of, 219-223, 220*t*
Exposure time, 14, 29-30, 272
  milliamperage and, 55, 56
  pediatric chest, 250
Extrapolation, exposure technique charts and, 224

F

Far-distance decentering, 125-126, 126
Feedtray, 169, *170*

Fiberglass casting materials, exposure factor
  selection for, 255
Field size, limiting, to image receptor size, 111
FIFO; *see* First in/first out
15% rule, kilovoltage and, 59, 60
Filament, cathode and, 14, *15*
Filament current, 23
Film
  blue-sensitive, 141-142
  characteristics of, 141-144, 202-210
  composition of, *137*
  construction of, 136-138, *137*
  direct-exposure, 140
  double-emulsion, 136, 140, *140*
  green-sensitive, 142
  orthochromatic, 142
  radiographic, 136-144
  screen, *140*, 140-141
  single-emulsion, 140, *140*
  types of, 140-141
  unexposed, storing, 182
Film contrast, 67, 68, 141, *142*, 205, 206
  average gradient and, 208
  exposure latitude and, 209
  maximum, 211-212, *212*
  slope and, 206
Film-handling areas, 182-184
Filmless cassette, 272
Film orientation for proper replishment, 175, *176*
Film processing, radiographic density and, 66
Film-screen contact, 154
Film-screen speed
  mAs and, 63
  radiographic density and, 63-64
Film-screen speed conversion formula, 63
Film-screen systems, interchangeability of,
  automatic exposure control and, 234-235
Film speed, 141, *142*, 202-205
  formula for, 204-205
  optical density and, 202
  speed exposure point and, 203
Filter
  safelight, 142-143, 183
  special, *35*, 35
Filtration
  added, 33, *34*
  beam, 32-35, *34*

Filtration—cont'd
  inherent, 33
  total, 33-34
First in/first out (FIFO), 182
Fixed kVp/variable mAs technique chart, 219-220,
  222-223, *222t*, 225
Fixer chemicals, solvent and, 167
Fixer tank, 169
Fixing, 166-168
Fixing agent, 166-167, *168t*
Flood replenishment, 176-177
Fluorescence, 3, 9, 145
Fluoroscopy, digital, *270*, 270-271
Focal distance, 116, 117
Focal range, 116, *117*
Focal spot, 17
Focal spot size, 79, 79-80, *80*
Focal track, 17, 18
Focused grid distance decentering, 125-126
Focused grids, 115, *115*, *116*, *117*
  upside down, 123, *124*
Focusing cup, cathode and, 14
Fog, 46
  chemical, 165
Foreshortening, 93, *93*
Frequency, 6, 7-8, *8*
Front screen of intensifying screen, 146

G
Gamma, 7, 208
GBX filter; *see* Green-blue x-ray filter
GCF; *see* Grid conversion factor
Generator output, 66, 265
Generator type, exposure factor modification and,
  265, 265-266, *266t*
Geometric properties, radiographic image quality
  and, 52, *52*, 78-96
Geometric unsharpness, 79, *79*, 83, 84
Glutaraldehyde, 166, *166t*
Gradient, average, *206*, 207-208
Gradient point, 207, 208
Graphite, target of rotating anode tubes and, 15
Green-blue x-ray (GBX) filter, 143, 183
Green-sensitive film, 142
Grid cap, 118
Grid cassette, 118
Grid construction, scatter control and, *113*, 113-118

Grid conversion chart, 62
Grid conversion factor (GCF), 119, 120
Grid cutoff
    distance decentering and, 125-126, *127*
    focal distance and, 117
    grid ratio and, 123
    lateral decentering and, 123-125, *124, 125, 126*
    scatter control and, 122-126, *127*
    types of, 123-126, *127*
    upside down, 123, *124*
Grid focus, scatter control and, *115*, 115-118, *116, 117*
Grid frequency, 113
Grid pattern, scatter control and, *114*, 114-115
Grid performance, scatter control and, 119-122
Grid ratio, 62, 113, *113*, 121
    decreasing, 122
    grid cutoff and, 123
    kVp and, 129
    patient dose and, 122
    radiographic contrast and, 114
    radiographic density and, 119
Grid selection, 118
Grid use, scatter control and, 128-129, *129t*
Grids, 102, 120, 131
    circular, 119
    focused, 115, *115, 116, 117*, 123, *124*
    linear, 114, *114*
    moving, scatter control and, 128
    nonfocused, 115, *115*
    off-level, 123-124, *124*, 125
    parallel, 115, *115, 116*
    radiographic, scatter control and, *112*, 112-113
    radiographic contrast and, 73, *73*
    radiographic density and, 62-63, *62t*
    reciprocating, 128
    scatter control and, *112*, 112-113
    types of, scatter control and, 118-119
    typical, 118
    wafer, 118
Guide plates, automatic processor and, 171, *172*
Gurney-Mott theory of latent image, 138, 162, *163*

H

Habitus, body, exposure factor modification and, *257-258*, 257-259

Halation, 140-141
Half-value layer (HVL), 34
Hardener
    developing and, 165-166
    fixing and, 167
Heat, 14
    darkrooms and, 184
    target of rotating anode tubes and, 15, 16-17
Heat unit (HU), 35-36
Hertz (Hz), 6
High contrast, 67
High frequency generator, 265, *265*
High-contrast film, 141
High-speed Bucky, 128
Hip radiograph, *154*
HIS; *see* Hospital information systems
Histogram, 275-277, *278*
Hospital information systems (HIS), 288
HU; *see* Heat unit
Humerus radiograph, *254*
Humidity, storage of unexposed film and, 182
HVL; *see* Half-value layer
Hydroquinone, 164, 165, *166t*
Hypersthenic type of body habitus, 257-259
Hyposthenic type of body habitus, 257-259
Hz; *see* Hertz

I

IF; *see* Intensification factor
Image acquisition, computed radiography and, 275, *276, 277*
Image brightness, window level and, 284
Image density, 46
Image display, computed radiography, 278-282
Image noise, 153
Image quality, matrix size and, 275
Image receptor contrast, 67, 68
Image receptor size, limiting field size to, 111
Image receptor unsharpness, radiographic image quality and, 85, *86*
Image receptors, 42, 134-159
    cassettes and, 155-157
    intensifying films and, 144-155
    radiographic film, 136-144
Imaging plate (IP), 272
Immersion heater, 179, *179*

Immersion heater coil, *179*
Inadequate processing, 181, 181*t*
Inherent filtration, 33
In-line heat exchanger, 180
InSight Thoracic Imaging System, *143*, 144
Instantaneous load tube rating chart, 36, *37*
Insulating oil, x-ray tube and, 18
Intensification factor (IF), screen speed and, 148
Intensifying screens, 144-155, *145*
    asymmetric, 144
    characteristics of, 146-153
    construction of, 145-146, *146*
    cross-section of, *146*
    maintenance of, 153-157, *156*
    purpose and function of, 144-145, *145*
    speed of, 85, 147-153, *152*, 152*t*
Intensity, 104, 194
Interchangeability of film-screen systems, automatic
    exposure control and, 234-235
Interspace material, 113
Inverse square law, 60
Invisible image, 48
Involuntary unsharpness, 87
Ion chamber, 233
Ionization, 43
Ionization chamber
    automatic exposure control and, 232, 233-234, *234*
    function of, 234
Ionization chamber AEC devices, 233
Ionizing radiation, darkrooms and, 183-184
IP; *see* Imaging plate

K

Kidney, ureter, and bladder (KUB) examination, 121
Kilovoltage (kV), 27-28, 272
    automatic exposure control and, 239, *240*
    beam penetrability and, 28
    changing, to compensate for pathologic
        conditions, 261, *262*
    15% rule and, 59, 60
    pediatric chest radiographs and, 350
    radiographic contrast and, 70, 285
    radiographic density and, *58*, 58-60, *59*
    scatter radiation and, 71
    speed of electrons and, 28
    x-ray quality and, 28

Kilovoltage peak (kVp), 9, 14, 58, 105, 129
Knee radiograph, 129
KUB examination; *see* Kidney, ureter, and bladder
    examination
kV; *see* Kilovoltage
kVp; *see* Kilovoltage peak

L

Lack of calibration, automatic exposure control
    and, 236
Lambda, 6
Laser camera printing, computed radiography
    and, 282
Last in/last out (LIFO), 182
Latent image, 48, 162
Latent image centers, 138-139
Latent image formation, 138-139, *139*
Lateral decentering grid cutoff, 123-125, *124*,
    125, *126*
Leakage radiation, x-ray tube and, 18
LIFO; *see* Last in/last out
Light emission, screen speed and, 148
Light transmittance
    formula for, 197
    optical density and, 197*t*, 198
Line focus principle, 31, *32*
Linear grid, 114, *114*
Loading charts, 36, *37*
Log of relative exposure, sensitometric curve and,
    199-200, *200*
Logarithmic scale, 197
Long-scale contrast, 67
Low contrast, 67
Low-contrast film, 141
Low-energy photons, *33*
Low-vacuum tubes, 3, 4
Lumbar spine radiograph, *252*, *255*
Luminescence, intensifying screens and, 145

M

mA; *see* Milliamperage
Magnetic resonance imaging (MRI), 270,
    288
Magnification
    calculation of, 90, *91*
    radiographic image quality and, 88-93

Magnification factor (MF), 90, 92
Manifest image, 48, 138, 162
mAs
   automatic exposure control and, 244
   part thickness and, 64
   quantity of radiation and, 55
   radiographic image quality and, 57
   source-to-image receptor distance and, 61
mAs conversion formula for screens, 149
mAs readout, automatic exposure control and, 243-244
mAs/distance compensation formula, 61
Mathematical Application for MF, 92
Mathematical formulas, 277-278
Matrix, computed radiography and, 273, *273,*
   274, 275
Matter, x-ray interaction with, 46
Maximum film contrast, 211-212, *212*
Measuring recorded detail, radiographic image
   quality and, 85-86, *86*
Media, contrast; *see* Contrast media
Medicine, nuclear, 270
Metallic replacement, 185
Metallic silver, developing and, 163-164
MF; *see* Magnification factor
Microswitches, 173-174, *174,* 175
Milliamperage (mA), 14, 29, 272
   automatic exposure control and, 239, *240*
   exposure time and, 55, 56
   and time, 30
Milliampere, 25, 29
Millimeters of aluminum (mm-Al), 34
Minimum response time, automatic exposure
   control and, 235
Minus-density artifacts, 185, *186, 188, 189*
mm-Al; *see* Millimeters of aluminum
Moisture, archival quality and, 180
Molybdenum, target of rotating anode tubes and,
   15, 16
Motion
   automatic exposure control and, 235
   elimination of, 88
Motion unsharpness, radiographic image quality
   and, *87,* 87-88
Motor drive, processing systems and, 171-173
Moving grids, scatter control and, 128
MRI; *see* Magnetic resonance imaging

N
Nature, 5
Near-distance decentering, 126
Neck radiograph, *263*
Negative contrast media, 77, *77,* 264
Neon-helium laser beam, *276*
Network systems, 288
Noise
   computed radiography and, 286-287
   image, 153
Non-Bucky studies, automatic exposure control
   and, 243
Nonfocused grids, 115, *115*
Nonscreen film, 140
Nuclear medicine, 270

O
Object size, determining, 92
Object-to-image receptor distance (OID), 74, 82
   air gap technique and, 130
   radiographic contrast and, 74, *74-75, 83*
   radiographic image quality and, 88-90, *89, 91*
OD; *see* Optical density
Off-level grid, 123-124, *124,* 125
OID; *see* Object-to-image receptor distance
Oil, insulating, x-ray tube and, 18
Optical density (OD), *196,* 196-199, 200, *211*
   diagnostic range and, 199
   film speed and, 202
   light transmittance and, 197*t,* 198
   sensitometry and, 210-211, *211*
Orthochromatic film, 142
O-shell, 164
Osteomyelitis, 259, *261*
Oxidation
   aerial, 173
   preservative and, 165
   use, 173

P
PA chest radiograph; *see* Posteroanterior chest
   radiograph
PACS; *see* Picture archival and communication
   systems
Pair production, 45
Pall Mall Gazette, 5

Parallel grids, 115, *115, 116*
Part thickness
   mAs and, 64
   measurement of, 218
   radiographic density and, 64
Particle concept of, 6
Pathologic conditions, exposure factor modification and, 259-262, *260t, 261, 262*
Patient, automatic exposure control and, 242-243
Patient dose
   collimation and, 103
   low-energy photons and, 33
   screen speed and, 148, *152t*
Patient exposure, screens and recorded detail and, 145
Patient motion; *see* Motion
PBLs; *see* Positive beam-limiting devices
Pediatric chest exposure time, 250, 251
Pediatric patients, exposure factor modification and, 250-251, *250t, 251t*
Pediatric skull radiography, 251
Penetrometer, *194, 195, 195*
Phantoms, radiographic, exposure technique charts and, 223-224
Phenidone, 164, 165, *166t*
Phosphor
   computed radiography and, 275
   intensifying screens and, 144, *147t*
   screen speed and, 150-151
   types of, 146-147, *147t*
Phosphor layer of intensifying screen, 146
Phosphorescence, 145
Photodisintegration, 45
Photoelectric effect, 10, 43, *44*
Photoelectron, 43
Photographic properties, radiographic image quality and, *52, 52-78, 95t*
Photography, 5
Photomultiplier tube (PMT), 275, 277
   automatic exposure control and, 232
   systems of, automatic exposure control and, 232-233, *234*
Photon absorption, 43
Photons, 8
   low-energy, *33*
   number of, quantum mottle and, 287

Phototiming, automatic exposure control and, 232
Physics, wave concept of, 6
Pick-ups, automatic exposure control and, 232
Picture archival and communication systems (PACS), 288
Pixel, computed radiography and, 273, *273, 274, 277*
Pixel number and spatial detail, 283
Plaster casts, exposure factor selection for, 255, *256*
Plus-density artifacts, 185, *186, 187*
PMT; *see* Photomultiplier tube
Pneumonia, 259, *261*
Polyenergetic x-rays, 32
Positions, exposure factor modification and, 251-255, *252, 253, 254*
Positive beam-limiting devices (PBLs), 111
Positive contrast media, 76, *76-77*, 263-264
Posteroanterior (PA) chest radiograph, 237, *238*
Postprocessing image enhancement, 273
Potassium alum, 167, *168t*
Potassium bromide, 165, *166t*
Potter, Hollis, 128
Potter-Bucky diaphragm, 128
Prep button, x-ray exposure and, 23, 24, *25*
Preservative
   developing and, 165
   fixing and, 167
Printing, laser camera, computed radiography and, 282
Processing, radiographic; *see* Radiographic processing
Processing cycle, 162
Processor
   automatic; *see* Automatic processor
   cold-water, 179
Processor capacity, 162
Processor dryer system, *180*
Projections, exposure factor modification and, 251-255, *252, 253, 254*
Protective layer of intensifying screen, 146

Q

Quality control, processing, 184
Quantum (quanta), 8
Quantum mottle, 153, *154*, 286-287

R

Radiation, 1-11
  discovery of, 1-11
  electromagnetic, 2, 6
  ionizing, darkrooms and, 183-184
  properties of x-rays, 9-10
  quantity of, mAs and, 55
  scatter; *see* Scatter radiation
  transmitted, 46-48, *47*
  x-rays as energy, 6-9
Radiation Control for Health and Safety Act of 1968, 111
Radiation exposure, intensity of, 194
Radiation-measuring devices, 232
Radiograph
  of abdomen, *75*, 264
  ankle, *253*
  anteroposterior, 65, 243, 251-253, *252, 253, 254, 254*
  archival quality of, 168, 169, 180
  cervical spine, *130*
  chest; *see* Chest radiograph
  first, 4
  hip, *154*
  humerus, *254*
  knee, 129
  lumbar spine, *252, 255*
  neck, *263*
  repeating, because of density errors, 57
  of sinuses, *109*
  storing, 183
  thoracic spine, 65
  unacceptable, calibration and, 236
  wrist, *253*
Radiographer, 10, 14
Radiographic artifacts, 185, *186t-187t, 188t-189t*
Radiographic contrast, 66-78, 205-208, *206*
  automatic exposure control and, 239, *240*
  controlling factors in, 70-72, *71, 72*
  factors in, 68
  influencing factors in, 73-78
Radiographic density, 53-66, 165
  controlling factors of, 54, 55-57, *56, 57*
  influencing factors of, 54, 57-66
Radiographic film; *see* Film

Radiographic film boxes, information found on outside of, 182
Radiographic grids; *see* Grids
Radiographic images, 138
  differential absorption and, 42-48
  formation of, 40-49
  geometric properties of, 78-96
  photographic properties of, 52-78
  quality of, 50-98
  sharpness of, 78-96
Radiographic phantoms, exposure technique charts and, 223-224
Radiographic processing, 160-191
  automatic processing equipment, 162, *164*
  film-handling areas, 182-184
  inadequate, 181
  purpose of, 162, *163*
  quality control and, 184
  radiographic artifacts and, 185, *186t-187t, 188t-189t*
  silver recovery and, 184-185
  stages of, 162-169
  systems of, 169-181
Radiographic quality, exposure technique charts and, 216
Radiography
  anatomically programmed, 244, *244*
  computed; *see* Computed radiography
  conventional
    computed radiography versus, 271-273, *272*
    limitations of, 271
  direct, computed radiography and, 287-288
  pediatric skull, 251
Radiology information system (RIS), 288
Radiowaves, 7
Rare earth elements
  intensifying screens and, 146-147
  screen speed and, 150-151
Ratio, grid; *see* Grid ratio
Reciprocating grids, scatter control and, 128
Reciprocity law, radiographic density and, 66
Recirculation system, radiographic processing and, *177*, 177-178, *178*
Recorded detail
  screen speed and, *152t*, 153
  sharpness and, 78-88

Reducing agents, developing and, 164-165
Reflecting layer of intensifying screen, 146, *152*
Regions, sensitometric curve and, 200-202, *201*
Relative exposure, log of, 199-200, *200*
Relative speed (RS), 63, 149
Replenishment
    processing systems and, 173-177, *174, 175, 176*
    solution performance and, 173
Resolution
    computed radiography and, 282-287
    measurement of recorded detail and, 85-86
Resolution grid, 85, *86*
Restrainer, developing and, 165
Revolutions per minute (RPM), 15
Rhenium alloy, target of rotating anode tubes
    and, 15
RIS; *see* Radiology information system
Roentgen, 6
Roentgen, Anna Bertha, 4, *4*
Roentgen, Wilhelm Conrad, 2, *2*
Roentgenology, 6
Roentgen rays, 6
Rotating anodes, 17-18
Rotating target, anode and, 15, *16, 17*
Rotor, anode and, 15, *16*
Rotor button, x-ray exposure and, 23, 24, *25*
RPM; *see* Revolutions per minute
RS; *see* Relative speed

S

Safelight filters, 142-143, 183
Safelights, darkroom and, 183
"Salt and pepper look," quantum mottle and, 153
Scale, logarithmic, 197
Scatter control, *73*, 100-133
    air gap technique and, 129-131
    beam restriction and scatter radiation, 103-105
    beam-restricting devices and, 102-103
    grid construction and, 113-118
    grid cutoff and, 122-126, *127*
    grid performance and, 119-122
    grid use and, 128-129
    moving grids and, 128
    radiographic grids and, 112-113
    type of beam-restricting devices, 105-111
    types of grids and, 118-119

Scattering
    beam attenuation and, 44-45, *45*
    classic, 45
    coherent, 45
    x-ray beam, 44
Scatter radiation, 46-48, *47*
    collimation and, 104
    image quality and, 113
    kilovoltage and, 71
    radiographic contrast and, 75
Screen film, *140*, 140-141
Screen leg, 145
Screen speed, 152*t*
    density and, 149
    selection of, 150
Screens, intensifying; *see* Intensifying screens
Secondary electron, 44
Sensitivity specks, 138-139, *139*
Sensitometer, 195, *195*
Sensitometric curve, 141, *142*, 199-202, *200, 203,*
    204, 231
    position of, along x axis, 203
    slope of, 205, 206
Sensitometric strip, 195
Sensitometry, 141, 192-213
    in calculation of exposure technique changes, 205
    clinical considerations of, 210-212
    definition of, 194
    equipment for, 194-196
    film characteristics of, 202-210
    optical density, 196-199
    sensitometric curve and, 199-202
    use of, 194
Sensors, automatic exposure control and, 232
Shape distortion, radiographic image quality and,
    93, 93-96, *94*, 95*t*
Sharpness
    radiographic image quality and, 78-96
    of recorded detail, 52
Short-scale contrast, 67
Shoulder region, sensitometric curve and, *201*,
    201-202
SID; *see* Source-to-image receptor distance
Silver (Ag), 138
Silver bromide (AgBr), 136, 138, *139*
Silver halide, 136, *137*, 138, *139*, 141, 163-164

Silver iodide (AgI), 136, 138, *139*
Silver recovery, 184-185, 185
Silver recycler, 185
Sine wave, 6, *8*
Single-emulsion screen film, 140, *140*
Single-exposure rating charts, 36
Single-phase generator, 265, *265*
Sinuses, radiograph of, *109*
Size distortion, radiographic image quality and, 88-93
Skull, pediatric, radiography of, 251
Slope
  and film contrast, 206
  of sensitometric curve, 205, 206
SOD; *see* Source-to-object distance
Sodium carbonate, 165, 166*t*
Sodium sulfite, 165, 166*t*, 167, 168*t*
Soft tissue technique, exposure factor modification and, 262-263, *263*
Solarization, 202
Solvent
  developing and, 166, 166*t*
  fixing and, 167, 168*t*
Sonography, 270
Source-to-image receptor distance (SID), 60, 111
  altering, between 40 and 72 inches, 61
  radiographic density and, 60
  radiographic image quality and, 81, *82*, 90, *91*
Source-to-object distance (SOD), 90
Space charge, 24
Space charge effect, 24
Spatial detail, pixel number and, 283
Spectral emission, 142, 143
Spectral matching, 142, 147
Spectral sensitivity
  radiographic film and, 141-143
  spectral emission and, 143
Speed
  of electrons, kilovoltage and, 28
  film, 141, *142*, 202-205
  of intensifying screens, 85, 147-153, *152*, 152*t*
Speed exposure point, 202-204, *203*, *204*
Speed point, 202, *203*, *204*
Splints
  exposure factor modification and, 255, 256
  exposure factor selection for, 256

Squeegee effect, automatic processor and, 171
Standby control, automatic processor and, 173
Stationary target, anode and, 15, *16*
Stator, anode and, 15, 16
Step-wedge densities, *69*, 195, *195*
Sthenic type of body habitus, 257-259
Storage
  of radiographs, 183
  of unexposed film, 182
Straight-line region, sensitometric curve and, 201, *201*
Subject contrast, 67, 68
Subtraction, computed radiography and, 278, *279*
Sulfite, 165, 167
Superadditivity, developing agents and, 165
Supercoat, radiographic film and, 136

T
Tabular grain (T-grain) technology, 137, *137*
Tanks, processing systems and, 169
Target, anode and, 15
Target interactions, 19-21
Technique charts, 217
  contents standardized in, 219
  exposure; *see* Exposure technique charts
  fixed kVp/variable mAs, 219-220, 222-223, 222*t*, 225
  limitations of, 217
  variable kVp/fixed mAs, *219-220*, 220-222, 221*t*
Technique overload, 36
Temperature
  developer, radiographic quality and, 178, 180
  storage of unexposed film and, 182
Temperature control, radiographic processing and, 178-180, *179*, *180*
T-grain technology; *see* Tabular grain technology
Thermionic emission, 23, 24
Thiosulfate, 168
  fixing agent and, 166
  washing process and, 167
Thoracic spine radiograph, 65
Three-phase generator, 265, *265*
Time
  backup; *see* Backup time
  exposure, 14, 29-30, 250
  milliamperage and, 30

Toe region, sensitometric curve and, 201, *201*
Total filtration, 33-34
Transmission, beam attenuation and, 45, *46*
Transmittance, light; *see* Light transmittance
Transmitted radiation, 46-48, *47*
Transport rollers of automatic processor, 170-171, *171*
Trough filter, 35, *35*
Tube current, 25, 26
  exposure time and, 30
  milliamperage and, 29
Tube filtration, radiographic density and, 66
Tube rating charts, 36, *37*
Tungsten
  target of rotating anode tubes and, 15, 16, 23
  x-ray tube and, 18
Turnaround rollers of automatic processor, 171, *171*

U

Unacceptable radiographs, calibration and, 236
Unexposed film, storing, 182
Unsharpness
  geometric, 79, *79*, 83, 84
  image receptor, 85, *86*
  object-to-image receptor distance and, 82
  resulting from patient motion, 87
  source-to-image receptor distance and, 81
Upside down focused grid cutoff, 123, *124*
Upside down focused grids, grid cutoff and, 123, *124*
Use oxidation, 173

V

Variable kVp/fixed mAs technique chart, 219-222, *221t*
Vertical transport system, processing systems and, 169-171, *170, 171, 172*
Video monitor, computed radiography and, 278-282, *279, 280, 281,* 283
Visibility factors, radiographic image quality and, 52-78
Visibility of recorded detail, 52
Visible image, 48
Voltage ripple, 265, 266
Voltage wave forms, 265, *265*

Voluntary unsharpness, 87
Voxel, computed radiography and, 273, *273*

W

Wafer grid, 118
Wash tank, 169
Washing, fixing and, 167-168
Water, 166*t*, 167
Wave concept of physics, 6
Wavelength, 6, 7-8, *8*
Wedge filter, 35, *35*
Window level and image brightness, 284, *284*
Window width, radiographic contrast and, 285, *285, 286, 286*
Wire mesh test tool, film-screen contact and, *155,* 156
Wratten 1A safelight filter, 143
Wratten 6B safelight filter, 143, 183
Wrist radiograph, *253*
Würzburg Physico-Medical Society, 5

X

X axis, position of sensitometric curves along, 203
X-radiation; *see* X-rays
X-ray beam attenuation, 43-48
X-ray beam scattering, 44
X-ray button, x-ray exposure and, 23, 27
X-ray emission spectrum, 22-23, *23*
X-ray exposure, 23-26, *24, 25, 26,* 27
X-ray photon absorption, 43
X-ray quantity, 30
  exposure time and tube current and, 30
  milliamperage and, 29
X-rays, 12-39
  anode heel effect and, 31-32, *33*
  beam filtration and, 32-35
  characteristics of, 10
  density of, 230, 231
  discovery of, 1-11
  dual nature of, 6
  emission spectrum of, 22-23
  as energy, 6-9, *7, 8*
  exposure to, 23-26, 27, 230, 231
  heat units and, 35-36
  interaction of, with matter, 46
  line focus principle and, 31, *32*

X-rays—cont'd
  naming of, 4
  polyenergetic, 32
  production of, 14-19, 20
  properties of, 9-10
  quality and quantity of, 26-30
  target interactions, 19-21, *22*
  tube rating charts and, 36, *37*

X-ray tube, 14, 18, *19*
  energy conversion in, 26
  extending life of, 36-38, *38*
  recent innovations in, 18-19
X-ray tube housing, 18, *19*

Z
Zero-crossover technology, 146